Struck by Hope

The True Story of Answering
God's Call and the Creation of
Little Pink Houses of Hope

Jeanine Patten-Coble

For more information and further discussion, visit

LittlePink.org and PattenCoble.com

Cover design by
Rick Nease
www.RickNeaseArt.com

Cover photo by
Daniel Pullen
www.DanielPullenPhotography.com

Published by Read the Spirit
Publishing services by Front Edge Publishing, LLC

For information about customized editions, bulk purchases or
permissions, contact Front Edge Publishing, LLC at
info@FrontEdgePublishing.com

When life gets tough,
I close my eyes,
spread my arms out and fall back
into the pillow of all of the people who love me

~ unknown

This book is dedicated to everyone who has been a part of my pillow throughout the years. It is written with the recognition that my father Larry Patten's influence on my life lives on long after his last breath. It is in honor of the devotion of my husband, Terry, who has always been walking beside me holding my hand, even when we have been a million miles apart. It is the culmination of many quiet hugs and the belief in my goodness from my son, Jake. There are numerous people who have challenged me, held me, and made me into a better person than I ever imagined. Because of each of you,
I have been changed for good.

Contents

Praise for
Struck by Hope

Struck by Hope is Jeanine's amazing journey of finding herself, finding God, and finding her purpose and passion when faced with breast cancer. It inspires the reader to listen and follow the calling of God, in order to truly live the life God has designed and prepared for them!

Maimah Karmo
Author of *Fearless: Awakening to my Life's Purpose Through Breast Cancer*, Founder of Bliss Magazine, CEO of Tigerlily Foundation

Struck by Hope had me at hello. It's rare to come across a gem such as this that provides inspiration amidst the reality that we each have faults and challenges all the while entertaining. This book is a spectacular reminder of a God who pursues and wants each of us as we are. Jeanine is an amazing example of faith and the impact it can have on the world and *Struck by Hope* provides a front row seat to the journey.

Heather Jose
Author of *Every Day We Are Killing Cancer*
Founder of Go Beyond Treatment

Struck by Hope is more than a book title; it's a calling to a different way of living. Jeanine Patten-Coble points us to how to become ridiculously present with candor, wisdom, and courage. This deeply personal story is inspiring and yet practical; posing questions and offering challenges to be ridiculously present and to answer God's call to do ANYTHING that he asks.

Fil Anderson
Author of *Running On Empty*

Struck by Hope teaches us how to use one of the most powerful life-tools all of us need after a diagnosis of breast cancer and for anyone facing devastation of any kind. Jeanine has a special name for this life-changing tool. She calls it learning to be "ridiculously present" in our daily lives. By being "ridiculously present," we no longer are prey to our fears or to judgments and dramas of others but instead we can instantly tune into a higher power and wisdom (God) to guide us forward even when this guidance surprises us with a new direction. If I had to recommend just one thing for anyone facing a trauma or trying to make a life-saving decision, this is the tool (and prayer!) I would unequivocally advise to use. Being "ridiculously present" is how we are led into living an empowered and meaningful life after diagnosis or devastating news.

Give this book to yourself and pay it forward by gifting it to other breast cancer survivors. Let's start a movement, a new tribe of survivors, to be a Ridiculously Present Breast Cancer Thriver.

Beverly Vote
25 year breast cancer thriver and publisher of
The Breast Cancer Wellness Magazine

Chapter 1

I cheated on my first husband.

The reasons I could give to explain this behavior or the details of the affair would cause you to yawn or adversely to scream about what a young, entitled little twit I was at the time. My first husband was not a bad guy, not a cheater, not an abuser. He was a run-of-the-mill 22-year-old focused on his career, and neither of us had any idea how to be married. We played house for a year and from the outside everything looked fine. The little things that I didn't like about him I picked apart and made into big things. I made a mistake and cheated on him. I cheated because I was caught up in myself and was going to make sure that the life I wanted was not one that had to be waited for. I cheated because it was easier to move on and not look back than to take a cold, hard look at my behavior.

In college, I created an elaborate ruse to convince my parents that I had been mugged in order to get them to send me additional money. I was not a kid from a poor family. Rather, I was from a middle class family, who, without the other five siblings attending private schools and needing to be clothed and fed, probably would have been defined as upper middle class. The stories about how I blew through my money would not cause a yawn. In fact, they are pretty hilarious and involved a lot of stupid behavior that make for some good fodder of what not to do when you go away to college.

I lied because I did not want to disappoint my parents—or at least that is what I told myself at the time. In reality, I lied strictly because the process of owning up to my own mistakes, taking accountability, and looking inward at the changes that I needed to make was too overwhelming of a process. This type of reflection would have taken way too much time away from my busy social life and the belief that the world revolved around me.

I am a person who is broken. I am a person who is flawed. Like many people, I was a person who was getting in my own way of seeing how God was showing up in my life. It was hard for me to imagine how God would ever want to be a part of my life because I was taking up all the space in the room. I was a person who I thought was totally screwed.

Do you have events or decisions from your past that you regret?

Chapter 2

There are so many times in life that I have looked around and thought, "What if people find out?" What if they find out that I don't know as much as they think I do? What if they find out that I am not really qualified for the job I have? What if my child realizes that I am making up parenting as I go along? What if my spouse realizes that I am just going through the motions?

Then what?

This version of a life of questioning sits deeply recessed in the mind without a tremendous amount of power until it pushes itself to the surface, until we question if we are actually good enough for the people, situations, accolades, or joys around us. Why do we seem to get caught up in the idea of not being good enough? What is it that causes us to see ourselves as *less than* as opposed to *greater than* or *equal to* everyone else? Not that life should be a game of comparisons—in fact, exactly the opposite.

For the better part of my life, the thought of praying in public was pure and holy terror for me. The people who claimed to love God with every ounce of their soul seemed to have the perfect words. The words came from a place seemingly divine and heavenly, as if God was using them as His ventriloquist dummy to ensure they had all of the right words. The inadequacy of not knowing Bible verses or the sheer fear that if I opened my mouth to pray, someone would judge me and see or think that I was not good enough kept me from praying in public.

The other big reason was that I really didn't know what to say because I wasn't exactly sure who God was.

Every morning growing up, I woke, put on a green plaid uniform and went off to Catholic school. I was surrounded by nuns, priests, crosses, prayers, and lots of people who fit my ventriloquist dummy description. But I was not connected. They were just words to me that other people were saying. I attended a Catholic, Jesuit university in the Midwest and I had the same experience. My parents were the most lovey dovey—at the time I would've used the word 'embarrassing'—couple who would walk up and take communion together. They were on the Jesus train all the way and had bought adjoining seats with a view. My parents insisted their children attend Sunday mass every single week because the alternative was a big old sin. At a very young age, I found myself revolting against this idea that God would punish me for anything bad that I did.

Being surrounded like this, how did I not have the words, any words to say about God? If I didn't have the pious words, shouldn't I have had at least some hateful words? I should have at least been able to come up with something. Luckily, in this religious environment, I always had the rote prayers to fall back on—the "Our Father's" and "Hail Mary's" that I could recite to look like I fit in, even though I never gave a single thought to the words I was saying.

So, I did not pray in public. And that also meant that any prayer life was easily relegated to a series of prayers when things were bad. You know, the prayers where you make all of the promises to God.

"If you will do this, then I will do this …" or "If you give me this, I promise that I will never do that again …"

To pray any other time was foreign and scary, so it was easier to just go through the motions of looking like a person of faith.

As I grew up and started living life without the threat of a Sunday mass sin, I could still go to church on Sunday if I wanted, try to be a good person in the community, and if I did it just enough, no one would be the wiser. No one would see that I did not have what I thought they had—a real relationship with God.

That game worked for years until God decided to drastically shake up my life. So imagine my fear when I was profoundly called by God to start an organization to help breast cancer patients. The very first thing that came to my mind was that I was not good enough.

Was it really even God? He would not choose someone like me. He would look for someone "church-ier." My resume didn't stack up to be the "do-gooder" in the world. I didn't even have a background in business. I was a high school history teacher. I couldn't do math well. I had a litany of reasons to explain why he wouldn't choose me. I couldn't lead other people if I didn't know where I was going. And I definitely couldn't be in charge of a plan that God had put together. That was a recipe for failure for me, personally.

Without knowing what "everything" was, at the time I felt like I had everything to lose.

I struggled with how to answer His call because I would need to look at my faith straight in the face. To answer His call was to take a cold hard look at the good, the bad, and the ugly. And there seemed like there was plenty of ugly. I had been playing this game of being a checkbox Christian for so long, I didn't know how to do it any different. My definition of a checkbox Christian:

- I went to church when it was convenient
- I sang the songs
- I prayed the rote prayers
- I gave to the collection plate
- I even volunteered when it was convenient for me
- I sent my son to a private Christian school so he could learn about God

When God showed up with a plan that was not part of my checkboxes, the first thing that I did was run. I had lots of other things that I could do besides answer His call.

And I had the best excuse ever—I was just diagnosed with breast cancer and had miserable treatments, depressing doctor appointments and countless scans that took up most of my waking moments. No one would ever think poorly of me for not answering His call—heck, I was in a battle to save my life.

When a person is diagnosed with cancer or a terminal illness, they may also experience a crazy shift in how others view or talk about them. All of a sudden, people are calling them brave, so inspirational, so blah, blah, blah. I could run from God's calling without anyone ever knowing and people would still call me brave! What a deal!

But, do you know the silly thing about running and having no one else know? I knew. I knew the constant proddings, nudges, and sacred echoes I was experiencing.

I grew up in a house with five siblings and the running joke (even still at holidays) to my mother was, "Who is your favorite?" My mom would answer in a way that seemed too politically correct—she loved each one of us the way we needed to be loved and the most. As I have gotten older, I realize that God does exactly the same thing with each of us. My relationship with God will not look like someone else's. My relationship with God is unique because that is how He made me. I took too many years trying to become like other Christians so that I would fit in with them and not be found out. But really, as soon as I learned that I will always fit in with God, my life changed forever. My journey of faith is not about looking like anyone else's journey or becoming God's ventriloquism dummy, but it is a constantly changing relationship where I learn more and more about His love and my ability to live in a space of peace because of His desire to love me as I walk on His journey.

So how has my prayer life changed? I started out as a person that would run to the restroom and literally get physically sick if I had to pray in public, to a person that decided that the only way to get over that was to put it all in God's hands and remember that He thinks I am good enough. So I started to pray in front of others. I don't know (and kinda don't care) if it even sounds good. I am not doing it as a way to impress anyone else. I do it because I have learned that I love Him. I try to remember that if I truly believe that He can do anything, that includes helping me overcome my fears and giving me the words that I am meant to say. I will never be alone. I will NEVER NOT be good enough. I will always be enough in His eyes.

What do you do when God calls you and you don't think you are good enough?

In God's eyes, you are good enough.

Which means you can do anything that He asks.

What is He calling you to do?

Chapter 3

I was 39 years old when I was diagnosed with an aggressive form of breast cancer. The months leading up to my diagnosis, I had been struggling with gallbladder pain. Numerous visits to various doctors caused me to be weary of what steps and actions to take. It wasn't necessary to take action, but I felt horrible. I made a decision in April of 2009 to get healthy and change the situation. I began walking a couple of miles a day, I started eating better and subsequently started losing some weight. It was the healthiest I had felt in years. I was working a high pressure job with the state department of education that required me to travel roughly three hours every day to some of the lowest performing schools in the state and coach their teachers. I bought a convertible to make the drive less stressful. I had an 11-year-old son that was super busy with basketball, friends, and just being goofy. My husband was busy with his lawn care and landscaping business. We were on the go!

I had no time for cancer.

But cancer found me and decided that it was going to ravage my body.

Luckily, I can thank my Catholic education for finding my cancer. When I was in high school, a woman from the health center came and brought a set of rubber breasts on a board for us to feel to educate our class about breast health. With tons of giggles and under-the-breath snide comments from a group of 15-year-old girls, we listened to what she had to say. None of us were more embarrassed to be in the room than the nun who drew the short straw for it to be scheduled during her class. I don't remember much about her actual demonstration, but I remember pointedly what the nun said as I was filing out of her room as the bell rang. I was always an incredibly large-busted girl, even at a very young age. She grabbed my arm, waved her hand in front of my chest and said, "With a chest that big, you will be the one to get cancer." Yes, that is really what she said! Keep in mind that this was part of the same group of adults in my life who knew best, so I took it to heart. From that moment on, I started doing self breast exams. It was a seed that was planted—albeit a completely unscientific, unfounded seed, but one that stayed with me.

Routinely on June 1, 2009, I did my monthly self breast exam like I had on the first day of every month for over 20 years. It wasn't a matter of feeling something and thinking, "What is that?" Nope, I felt it and I knew immediately. It was huge, the size of a ping pong ball. Where had it come from? Last month's exam had revealed nothing at all. I sat and didn't want to go downstairs to let my husband know. Those few moments were mine. Those moments were the last that I had before I had to deal with anyone else's tears, emotions, or my own insecurities. I sat on the bed and said one of my prayers that I had grown easy with.

"God, if you will just let the doctors take care of this, I will do ANYTHING that you want. Just don't let me die!" I wonder if that day He said with a smirk on His face, "OK, I got the perfect "ANYTHING" for you. Get ready!"

Little did I know just how big of an anything He would ask.

The subsequent week in doctor's offices was a mere formality. I knew. My doctor knew. We were just waiting on someone to read a test. I started to tell family and friends about my appointments and the possibility of cancer to a litany of "I am sure that you will be fine. It is probably just a cyst," responses. Every conversation I had that week was to help prepare them, not me. I already knew.

My journal entry from the night before the results came in still captures that time period in a way that if I tried to put words to it now, years later, would not be able to recapture.

June 2009

In 24 hours, everything in my life could change. Well, not everything. My husband will remain the same wonderful man. My son will still adore me. My friends will still care about me. My parents will still love me unconditionally. What will change is that I could very easily become one of those people. One of the people that others show pity to and say my name and a weird phrase like "she was diagnosed with cancer, but she's such a good person." And I guess I should be happy that I think so highly of myself that I think people would finish that sentence with the good part.

What could possibly change? In less than 24 hours I am going to find out that I have breast cancer. Writing those words on the page just made my heart stop for a minute and almost made me cry.

I have decided that the way that I handle this from the very beginning will help to set the tone for the entire process—or more importantly, the way that people view me. I do not want to be a victim. I do not want this to define me. Truly, I do not want to have this because I do not want it impinging on my life.

There is a part of me, though, that has been preparing my whole life for this moment. When I was younger, I had this eerie feeling that I would not make it past my 39th birthday—it was always something about a big disease that would take me. I have had moments in the past six months when I have been thinking about my legacy, how I need to help prepare the people around me because something big is about to happen. That something big in my head was a brand new educational consulting business, NOT cancer! I guess my body got the wrong memo.

But I know what I want 24 hours from now.

I want…

Dignity

To continue to find joy all around me

To dance, dance, dance

To feel love, not pity

To marvel in the wonder that if I have cancer, God has given it to me as a gift. A gift that I might not understand, but one that will make me more of the person that I am supposed to be (that one was hard to write—do I even believe in God and would I still believe if He does this to me? What will I believe in 24 hours?)

To cross paths with the people who will help me see what I need to see

To be cared for by people that I trust

To learn to put this disease in a box so that it does not define me

To lose weight as a bonus

To get new boobs as an extra bonus

To laugh

For my husband to still look at me like he does

For my son not to let this affect his idea of how God might love him

To cry when I need to cry, yell when I need to yell, and curl up with I need to and then move the hell on

For people not to treat me like I am dying

To use this experience to make a difference

To LIVE.

In 24 hours the process will start. I want to be ready. But how can I be?

Have you ever been faced with a reality that you did not want to deal with?

Have you known that you were at a pivotal juncture in your life and tried to bargain with God?

Write out a list of what you want. Where does God fit in?

Chapter 4

The next part of the journey was going to be one of the hardest imaginable. Telling everyone about a diagnosis or that you may die is truly a form of torture for both parties. The person delivering the news wants so hard to put on a brave face, but the inside of your mind is on overdrive and your heart is full of fear and worry. You suddenly look at the people around you and see their pain so clearly. The pain in hearing the diagnosis and the pain they will feel if you don't make it. I never blamed myself for my cancer, but it is hard not to see that your diagnosis is the reason that others are hurting.

Your heart opens up in a way you never imagined because it needs the extra space to have pieces of it break and still remain beating.

And so the brave face dance begins.

The one where I put a brave face on for you, and you put one on for me, and what is lost is that I will never really know how anyone truly feels or reacts. They will save that for other people in their lives that will give them support because I am sick. As everyone tried to dance around with a brave face, I kept thinking about the one face on which I would see the gravity of feeling. The true, honest, real face of my son. The word "dread" does not even come close to explaining the feeling that I felt. How could I make something so enormous and painful bearable for my child? How can I be the person who takes away the luxury of his innocence that he will never get back? How can I expect an 11-year-old to deal with something that I have no idea how to deal with?

By sheer chance, our yearly vacation to the Outer Banks of North Carolina was scheduled the day after my biopsy. We had been traveling there for 15 years every summer. The same beach. The same week. The same house. No surprises. Until this year. This was the year that the trip to the beach was going to take on an all-new meaning, in more ways than one.

My husband and son climbed into the truck and I into my convertible. I was a woman on a mission not to cry while I was driving, but also determined to try to get emotion out along the way so that I could be strong for my son when we told him how our lives would be changing. That summer was filled with lots of great music, but the song that continued to come on at least a dozen times during the six-hour drive was *The Climb* by Miley Cyrus. That song was the audio equivalent of a Mack truck wreck. I simply couldn't look away! From my car's speakers, Miley kept reminding me that I would face one mountain after another, in life. And, even with the best of intentions, even with the greatest strength I could summon: *"Sometimes I'm gonna have to lose."* Whatever station was on the radio, that song kept returning, over and over and over again like endless punishment, reminding me: *"Sometimes I'm gonna have to lose."* Then came the song's reassurance: *"Ain't about what's waiting on the other side—It's the climb."*

So often throughout my long cancer journey, it was about the climb over one mountain after another. Frequently, I would find myself like this—in the quiet solace of the car listening to a song and crying. I would let myself feel all of the pain and worry about not making it. Solace is important. This is an incredibly difficult pain to share with another person, because then you have to deal with that person's feelings as well as your own. It is no longer about you. Those quiet moments were tortured and sad, but they were necessary for me to be authentic.

So with Miley Cyrus playing, me crying with the top down in my convertible and the tears all over the road, we made it to the beach house in the Outer Banks of North Carolina for the big conversation. I had thought about all of the words that we would say to try to make this unbearable reality easier for our son.

Then I looked at that little boy who was running about, excited to be at his favorite place in the whole world and couldn't do it. I decided I had to go for a run. I wasn't ready. Miley and I had been climbing and it was time to regroup and eliminate any of my own fears and issues for one of the most important conversations of my life.

And then it happened.

Chapter 5

The southern Outer Banks of North Carolina is a very desolate, beautiful place that calls for moments of solitude in its pounding surf. I knew that I needed to clear my head, so I went for a run on a road that I have walked down for over 15 years. Everything was ordinary. Everything was the same. Except this time, I went just a little bit farther down Old Lighthouse Road. As I was running, it came up in the distance. Here, right on the ocean was a compound of 43 houses with a chain link fence around it, completely abandoned. Not a soul in sight. I could see that this was a community at one time. There was a swing set and a playground in the middle. Where there once was life, now there were only houses that looked similar. Each had their own beating that it had weathered. I ran around the chain link perimeter, looking for any sign of what it was, to no avail.

Why in the world would there be so much beachfront, prime real estate abandoned?

Who would walk away and leave it for the fury of the ocean to tatter?

Why had I never known that it was here?

It piqued my interest and was a great distraction from the conversation that I should have been having in my head—the one where I pick all of the perfect words to tell my son that I might die. I was determined that I could win an Academy Award for motherhood if I just did this one thing right. I had made a lot of mistakes, but I could not mess this one up.

I turned to run back to our rental house and took about 15 steps on the road when I was hit.

My chest felt like it had been punched, but not in a way that hurt.

My brain had become completely free of the sad and crazy thoughts that had taken up prime real estate in it just minutes before. I found myself inexplicably down on the ground and a reverberation in my heart that spoke very clearly. It carried tangible waves of sound, but the sound was coming through my soul to my brain.

I wasn't hearing a voice in my ears. I was struck by God's voice in my heart. His message was clear.

Create a place like this for cancer patients to be loved.

Again, a second time.

Create a place like this for cancer patients to be loved.

So clear with no other direction. God was being awfully vague. And in that moment, I knew that something big was getting ready to happen. But then I thought, are you kidding me?

I had just been diagnosed the day before. The day before! There was no way that God was talking to me. Faced with the complete fear of my diagnosis, I immediately panicked that the doctors had only been focusing on cancer in my breasts. One biopsy is all that they had done. The doctors hadn't performed any other tests or checked out the rest of my body. Clearly, the cancer wasn't just in my breast; it had travelled to my brain. There is no way that God would talk to me so clearly. Forget wondering if I was good enough or not, I had to get home and tell my husband that I am hallucinating, hearing voices, worrying about having a brain tumor or some other explanation that would make sense.

My husband was knee deep in his own game of trying to keep it all together that afternoon. He was in just as much pain as I was. My husband Terry is a solid, rock of a person. We live in the South and everyone would agree that he is a good ol' boy—one that would do anything for anyone. We had been married for years and he adored me and focused so much of his energy on being there for our son, Jake. He is the dad that went on all of the field trips and was front row at every basketball game. He was engaged in making sure that his family was happy, protected, and cared for. And all of a sudden, the diagnosis that had landed in our home was something that he could not fix.

When I came in from my run, I don't even know what he actually heard, except a frantic wife that had a story about hearing voices, which might possibly be just another way of putting off telling our son of the diagnosis. God had knocked very clearly and loudly—but the truth is, I was scared of it, so it was easy to let go of.

I had other things that were more important, or so I told myself. I wrote in my journal that night that I was scared, because if what had happened was real that "God just knocked the crap out of me." (Well, really I used a curse word.)

My husband, son, and I sat on the couch in our pajamas. The news of my diagnosis was coming out of left field, with no warning for our son. I can still remember every detail—what my son was wearing, what he was drinking, the look on his face and the moment that everything changed for him. When I told him that I had breast cancer, I could see his world stop.

He just stopped being happy in that moment.

I had never actually seen him not happy. I had seen him throw a fit to get what he wanted when he was little or get mad because he couldn't learn to do something right. But never a complete removal of happiness from his face. It's like his heart was talking to his skin and eyes and they were clearly in sync with the same sad message. One of the most difficult parts was that every time he started to cry, he would recoil and pull toward my husband. He knew where he needed to find solace in that moment, and it was not with the mother who had just devastated his world.

And then the question that I feared.

"Are you going to die?"

I couldn't swallow, I couldn't breathe. I couldn't lie to him. I reassured him that I was going to live with cancer, that I was not planning on dying from it and that we were a team that was going to fight together. We answered all of Jake's questions as best we could, not making any promises or creating any unnecessary fear. When he finally hugged me, I realized that I had never experienced the true joy of holding him until that moment. I thought that I had—when he was born, lying in his bed reading to him when he was little, holding him when he was sick, watching him play ... but none of those moments compared to the crying love of a boy in his boxers and T-shirt trying to hold on to the idea that his mom is going to have to fight to live. None of it compared to understanding that every hug moving forward might be limited.

It became crystal clear that there was no way that I was going to leave him. I was going to fight like you have never seen anyone fight before.

That week was riddled with crying, laughing, trying to have perfect moments, reveling in the broken moments, and learning to live with these weird cells that I could not feel physically, but were taking up too much residency in my brain.

I had spent the week thinking about my run and those abandoned houses in the back of my head. I was barely able to process how I would be able to handle over a year of chemotherapy and treatments and if I would survive, nonetheless some cockamamie calling from God. I couldn't fathom anything else on my plate.

I had a job.

I was a mom.

I was a wife.

I was busy.

It was time to just chalk the experience on my run up to just a crazy girl on an emotional day. I would not need to speak about it or tell anyone what had happened.

At the end of the week, Terry and I walked down the beach to the location of the Hatteras Lighthouse. He had asked me to marry him there, 13 years prior. (And yes, he is the man that I cheated with, and we are still together over 20 years later.) We stood on the beach and I let the tears flow on his chest. "We can make it through anything," he said. He was talking about the upcoming cancer treatments, the possible loss of my breasts, and the changes in every aspect of our day to day life.

And in the distance, over his shoulder, I could see the compound of houses staring at me. That word ANYTHING again. I had said my frantic desperate prayer of "*God if you fix this, I will do ANYTHING.*" Be careful when you say it, you never know what just might come about.

Are there times when you have felt compelled, nudged, or pushed to do something?

What would listening to that calling have looked like in your life?

How would you react if God called you to do ANYTHING today?

Chapter 6

I have looked back on that day at the compound so many different times and always circle back to the same amazing realization. On the absolute worst possible day in my life, the day that I dreaded telling our son about my cancer, God showed up. Not only did He show up, He knocked me over. If it had been a scene out of a cartoon, it would have been God with a big huge frying pan hitting me over the head, stars swirling around me.

God's calling can be big and powerful moments, faint voices, or small and tender nudges. It can be a voice in the darkness or a trumpet in the light. It is not about the calling, but about how you listen and choose to answer. He showed up, but I did not listen. I thought about listening, but did not answer His call because I did not think I was good enough for Him to choose me. If God is all knowing and all powerful, that means that He knows every bad thing that I ever did or thought and knows just what a hot mess I am on any given day. Nope. I could not do it.

It was also difficult because as I was going through treatment and there were so many unknowns about my health. My tumor initially grew even larger before I started chemotherapy. Taking the chemotherapy caused my heart to experience cardiotoxicity and it became a challenge just to walk up a flight of stairs. The treatments were doing a number on my ability to think clearly. Chemo brain is a very real phenomenon. I couldn't even imagine looking back at God's calling and having the energy or mental capacity to plan a meal, not to mention create a strategic plan for a brand new non-profit organization. Nope. I had every excuse in the book.

And then all of the little knocks started happening. When I look back at my life, I see all the other ways in which He had quietly tapped me to say, "I am here."

Why had I never given those small knocks any credence?

When I was 14 years old, I was headed to the Junior Olympics to play basketball in Walla Walla, WA. My team was from Pennsylvania and we each had to raise money to pay for our trip. I had tried to raise the money and came up $700 short. The day before the money was due, I walked out to the mailbox and opened it to find a plain white envelope with my name on it, with $700 inside. To this day, I have no idea where it came from. At the time, I was focused on trying to find out who would do such a thing rather than looking at how someone out there had been moved to act in such a way.

When I was in my 30s and struggling with endometriosis, I was on a plane headed to Rhode Island to visit my sister. I was distraught with constant pain that I could not seem to ever get relief from. I looked out the window of the plane to a beautiful blue sky and felt my shoulders relax and very clearly felt a presence on my shoulder. And a voice that said "I have you," which caused a total sense of calm in me. My pain subsided and became much more manageable.

Why did I gloss over these experiences, or think that they were all voices in my head, or just coincidences?

I think that there are barriers that I had built up that were hard to break down to be able to understand the clarity of my life and the way in which God could use me.

For most people, the barriers to not seeing Him are not easy to understand and can be a complicated, tangled web. Imagine a four-lane road with construction happening. There are cones, portions of one lane closed, even a bridge that is out. All of the people driving down the road have the same barriers, but what they are driving determines their journey. The man in the 18-wheeler has the ability to plow through the cones if he wants, but doesn't have the turning radius to pivot at the roundabout without taking out another car. The young girl on the bike can zig-zag in and out of the cones with ease and pass other cars that are stopped. She can ride along the shoulder of the road to avoid the traffic, yet she cannot do anything when she gets to the bridge that is out. And the woman in the minivan who feels like she's the last in line to get past every obstacle, waiting until everyone else gets out of the way, throws her hands up and decides to get off at the next exit to eliminate any further headache. A barrier to one person may not even remotely be something that affects another person.

They can seem overwhelming. But the barriers are very real.

I wonder if the clarity that came with the cancer was a big reason that all of a sudden the knocks and nudges seemed like they belonged to God for the first time.

The week after I was diagnosed was no better than the first. In fact, much more grave. After getting home from the beach, we woke the next morning to a call from the assisted living facility where my mother-in-law resided. They told us that she had suffered a brain aneurysm and had been taken to the emergency room. My mother-in-law died that day.

My own mother went to my oncology appointment with me later that week as my husband prepared for his own mother's funeral. The news was horrible, with facts and figures that I refused to accept. In hindsight, the grimness of the day and the doctor's ambivalence caused me to become my own advocate and find a different doctor that believed in healing not only my body, but caring for all aspects of me. But the day was unbelievably eye-opening in ways I had never imagined. As we left the doctor's office, I walked into the side parking lot that faced a small field.

And I cried.

I cried the ugly cry with snot coming from my nose and tears that won't quit. The kind where your mouth is so distorted because the pain you feel is wringing itself out of your body.

And then the clarity came. Not of the disease or my future, but the clarity of my surroundings. I was being bombarded with visual and auditory stimulus. It was like every single leaf on the tree I was sitting under had its own shape and definition and needed to be acknowledged as such. Every sound was crystal clear and competing with the others. I could feel the warm wind in a way that didn't make sense because it was barely moving. The best way to describe it is like in that brief instant, my life moved from a regular TV to the entire world becoming high definition.

So, not only did God start to become clearer, so did everything else.

I started noticing the intricacies of people and how they interact. I started seeing how people around me needed care. I started seeing the knocks as knocks and not just coincidences. I found myself being ridiculously present for the first time in my life.

I hadn't realized until I was faced with the idea that I might not make it, how much more present I could be with people. How little I had been present before. In my head, there were tons of conversations where I was already searching for a response or tuning the person out because what they were saying didn't interest me. I could sit in a room and not really take in another person's joy because I was too busy thinking about my to-do list for the week. When I was 'present,' it was because it was expected.

I realized through my cancer diagnosis that being ridiculously present was the only way in which I would now be able to live.

That clarity changed my life.

Now, some might say that I was searching for meaning in a world that seemed to be spinning out of control. I don't remember searching as much as I remember continually being slapped in the face. My father passed away from cancer some years ago and still to this day, I will be going along in my day when out of the blue, I have an emotional memory that hits me like a freight train going 1,000 miles per hour that takes me from a normal moment to one where I fall apart. It is that same sort of instantaneous shift that happened after I was diagnosed.

Where was it coming from and why was it attacking me? I wanted to scream, "I am sick, leave me alone!"

If I wasn't searching, then how was I able to start to hear His small voice?

Why could I not see His hand at work so many times in my life?

I think that it is because I just did not want to give God the credit. If I did, I would have to see that He might have plans for me. I might even have to figure out what I believe to be able to answer His call.

Have you been saying that you are waiting to hear God's plan for your life?

Are you searching or are you listening?

What do you need to do in your life to clear out the other noise so that you can listen?

Chapter 7

My biggest fear in answering God's call was worrying that what I believed would be put on display for everyone else to pick apart. They would see that I was flawed, broken, and a work under construction. They might judge me. Was I strong enough to handle that judgment? Would they even believe that God was talking to me, or even more dangerous, what if they were right and somehow it wasn't really God?

Leading up to this moment, I never had to worry about it because I had found a way to never really talk about my beliefs. I developed the best diversionary tactic to ward off any of the people that would profess their beliefs and try to question mine. I ran into them in college, in the workplace, within my own family, and in society as a whole.

Give me a dinner party with a Christian that wanted to say that if I didn't believe in Jesus, I wouldn't go to heaven, and it was on!

When I was in high school, I felt very jaded about the institution of the church. I felt like one particular priest in the parish always focused on how much everyone should give to the offering plate. It drove me nuts! It seemed like he was focusing on the wrong thing. Granted, I could not have told you what he should have focused on, but I had my one thing to complain about. And I hung onto it. I told my parents that I wanted to find a different Catholic church to attend, maybe one down by the university that might better meet my needs. Keep in mind that my needs at the time were for a Church to believe what I believed, because I knew it all.

So off I went.

At first I was content to go. Just the plain difference of having a guitar over a stodgy old organ seemed better. But then it started again. I would find something that didn't quite fit my needs. This went on for the better part of my 20s and 30s at various denominations. I was like Janet Jackson walking into a new church, demanding the answer to the question, "What have you done for me lately?" It was all about me.

I didn't want to hear the teachings or the love that many of them tried to show. I listened to a sermon and picked it apart as I was listening. As a preacher was talking, I was already putting my argument together in my head. I was always ready to start a conversation about faith with, "You really want me to believe that ..."

I was a smart, college educated woman that could clearly see through any of the stuff that they were slinging at me every Sunday. I believed that I was smarter than them and had an incessant need to be right. I had a need for others to see my side, but I did not want to see theirs. I used my academic training in history to turn around Biblical stories and throw them back in an unwitting person's face. I cannot even begin to comprehend how many times I would say something like, "You mean to tell me that with all of the good in the world that Gandhi did, he will not be in heaven?" or "The story of Ishmael is essentially the story of Noah, but it happened thousands of years before the Bible was ever written, you expect me to believe that those are God's words?" Over and over again, put me in a room with a believer and I would systematically pick their faith apart, piece by piece. They had their beliefs and I had my facts. I could be tolerant of lots of other religions, but not Christians. I could be tolerant of other religions, but not the one in which I was raised. Something was off. I was an academic elitist who realized that if I kept slinging questions, insults, and logic at others, I never truly had to look at what I believed.

I was focused on what I believed about social issues, political ideologies, and bigotry, but not focused on what my soul actually believed.

And that is such an important statement. I never had to look at what I believed. I see that as such a prevalent aspect of our society today. I am not talking about science over faith, but rather the need to be right over the need to reflect on what barriers each individual throws up to protect himself or herself.

I had been surrounded in my early years by structures and processes of indoctrination. I had chosen in my teens to seek out something different and found nothing. I grew comfortable in my 20s and 30s, picking apart everyone else's faith, and I found myself unbelievably dumbfounded by the idea that I had spent my life searching for something, but never really asked myself the simple question, "At the core of your being, what do you believe?"

Figuring out what I believed was a place of total discomfort. There are parts of what I believe that go against beliefs instilled in me when I was growing up. Other aspects of what I believe are in direct contradiction to many of my siblings' beliefs, whom I love and respect.

Figuring out what I believed was a matter of surrendering to a quiet conversation that coexists between my soul and my heart.

After doing some work, if it ended up that I did clarify my feelings towards God, did I even want to be someone who talked about God and His impact on my life? The examples that I had around me were ones that either seemed weird and disconnected to the real world, or they seemed like the do-gooder perfect Christian that I would hate to be around. They could recite Bible verses like it was a competitive sport. They could pray and fill the room up with a bunch of people mumbling "amen …" "praise Jesus" or, "speaking in tongues." I was worried that after reflecting, listening, and doing some hard work, I would figure out what I believed, but still might not fit in anywhere.

God is not an issue, He is love. Remove social issues from your thinking. Remove politics from your thinking. Remove your own hurts from your past from your thinking. Who is God to you?

At the core of your being, what do you believe?

Chapter 8

The months following my diagnosis were a whirlwind. My days were filled with trying to have everything as normal as possible in a completely upside down world. There were events in the first six months after my diagnosis that caused me to be able to start hearing the knocks much more clearly, and it wasn't because life had become easy. On the contrary, it was a period of great struggle. Here is an abridged version of the first six months after my diagnosis during which I wondered if God had not received the memo that I had cancer:

- My husband Terry's mom died. We buried her the same day that a doctor told me I had a 25% chance of surviving one year.

- A cousin, just a few years older than me, died and left three beautiful kids without a dad. At his funeral, my grandmother told me she did not want me to be next. People really do say these things!

- I had relied upon my mom and dad to be there as I started chemo. My dad's heart had other plans. He had an aortic aneurysm and had surgery to put a pacemaker in—all while they were 600 miles away in Florida.

- My car was hit by a deer that did not have insurance.
- Once my car was fixed, it was then part of a hit and run accident on my birthday that left me bumperless.
- I was put in isolation at my cancer hospital for a week due to the possibility of shingles thanks to an inexplicable rash.
- All three kitchen appliances broke and needed to be replaced in the same week.
- A pipe burst, causing major water damage in our house, requiring us to completely replace an entire floor of our home and had us living with fans the size of refrigerators for a month.
- The day after all of the new electronics and furniture were delivered after the water damage remodel, we decided to go to the beach to get away and relax. We came home to a door that had been knocked in and all of our valuables stolen.
- All of the while, I was experiencing every single crazy side effect of the chemo treatments and felt like I was going to die.

In a world where I was questioning God anyway, I really felt like I was under attack and could barely handle anything more.

I found myself at the breaking point on a daily basis.

My health felt like it was deteriorating (even though my cancer was actually shrinking). I could tell my husband's heart was hurting tremendously—he couldn't stand to see the woman that he loved turning into a shell of a person who she once was. I couldn't imagine doing anything for anyone else because we could barely make it through a day without a catastrophe happening. But in each of these situations, when I found myself feeling like I was too weak, I had a sense that God was taking care of it. Not the auto insurance adjuster or the appliance shopping, but He was taking care of making sure that the right people were on my path.

He was caring for my soul so that it did not break.

He was waiting for me to walk through this so that I could walk with Him.

He was pursuing me and waiting for me to let Him catch me.

In short, He was waiting for me to say yes to what He had asked.

Deep in the recesses of my mind, I kept thinking that God had shown up in the biggest way possible, on the hardest day of my life, with the greatest mission I had never imagined and that something good could come from all of the strife, if I had the courage to let Him in.

In every single bad event that transpired in the first six months, each was accompanied by a slight nudge. People became more important. All of the material stuff became less important. It was my son, Jake, who on returning home from the beach to find our house had been robbed, caused me to lift my spirits and look at things differently.

We had pulled into the driveway and could tell that our back door had been smashed in. My son and I waited in the driveway as my husband checked the house and called the police. As we were standing in the driveway, side by side, he put his arm around me and said, "Our family does really good in the face of adversity." I don't know if I was more excited that he was able to see it so clearly, or because he, a sixth grader, had used the word adversity in a sentence correctly! And I just started to laugh and squeeze him a little harder. He was right. We had gotten through so much and we were able to see that we were still strong.

I could feel God's presence in his hug that day. I knew that I had been given every reason to turn away and walk away from God. I had every reason to blame Him for the misfortune of my disease and the previous six months of pain. I had every reason to say no.

But what would happen if I said yes?

It was at that point that I sat down and talked to Terry and Jake about the run on the beach and what I had been think-ing. This time, I wanted to hear what they had to say. I found myself talking about God in a way that I never had. "God has called me to do this ... I can feel God leading me to do this ... I don't know how to do it, but if we stick together, I think it can work ..." As the words were coming out, I felt like they were looking at me in a completely different way. A way that I wasn't sure that I liked.

These were the people closest to me and I couldn't imagine opening my heart up to God and letting them down in some way.

When I first told my mom that I felt like God was calling me to do this, I was taken aback by her initial response as well. She was the epitome of the faithful woman and her response, "Well, are you sure that it is God's voice and not your own?" took me completely off guard. It was my worst fear and it had happened the very first time I talked to someone who knew me really well, my own mother.

And there is was, my fear that people wouldn't believe me.

With my fear and insecurity raging, it seemed like my own mother couldn't imagine God thinking that I was good enough to choose either.

I even went to talk to my pastor about the calling to which I was being led. I set up the meeting, knowing that he would talk me out of it. My body had been ravaged by treatments and surgeries, I needed time to recover, not take on a monumental challenge. I was looking at the easy way out—one where I could get off the hook of having to take that cold hard look at my faith and answer God's call. In my mind, that was the space that I had lived in for so long. It was comfortable, at least I thought.

My pastor listened intently. I could see the smirk forming around his mouth. He leaned in with his grin and his eyes filled with excitement and called me out. He looked me squarely in the eyes, the kind of look that you can't look away from. "God called Moses to part the Red Sea and lead the people to Egypt. He didn't call anyone else. God doesn't call thousands of people to do His work and just hopes that one of them says yes," he said.

"He calls one person for one thing that He wants done in this world. He loves you. He called you. Why not you?"

No longer could I default to the idea that I am not good enough. No longer could I run and hide. How could a God to whom I felt so disconnected decide to show up and ask something of me? My life no longer made sense, because what He was asking was no longer about me. He was asking something huge. He was asking my entire life to be turned upside down. It was an invitation to be uncomfortable, to shackle my already-hurting family to a financial burden and change greater than I ever imagined. He was asking me to put myself out there and take a chance on Him.

He was asking me to believe that ANYTHING could happen.

He was asking me to put myself in a place of vulnerability and possible ridicule. In short, it was time to figure out who this God guy was and stop running. It was decision time. And so my journey of learning that I AM good enough started.

And the first thing that I had to accept was that I was His. This was the most difficult lesson of every lesson that I have learned. It seems like it should be the easiest, but in fact was the monumental first step for me in moving forward.

It was the first time since that day on the beach of the initial calling that I really put real words to God's plan. But the words took on a new meaning. My soul had decided that I would have to answer His call. I knew that it would create a whirlwind of other decisions that would change our lives and I was well aware that I might not live long enough to see it all through. But I had to do it. I had to say yes. If I didn't, there was no way that I would ever try again. I didn't think that God would ever try again with me. It was now or never.

Have you ever been in a season where life just seems like it is too much to handle?

Have you wondered where God is?

How would you have felt if you believed that He was still pursuing and chasing you and that He had not run away from you?

Chapter 9

Transformation began for me when I really looked at what I believed and started living an authentic life. But what actually is an authentic life? Living an authentic life starts when you believe that you are good enough.

Our society is very interesting. It seems like so many people, especially women, are plagued with feelings of not feeling good enough. Societal norms, expectations, and social value have created a world in which many females innately start from a place of not feeling good enough and work to build up to a standard of good enough that has never actually been set, making it impossible to reach. The gender roles that are pervasive in society play a hand in this sort of thinking as well. Just when I feel like I am good enough at my job, I feel not good enough as a mom. In an attempt to be the perfect mom, women can lose themselves and never feel like they are doing anything else right. This quest to be good enough is dominated by trying to compare oneself to some standard. I've found that there are four main categories that are pervasive in the trappings of not feeling good enough:

Not as good as the Joneses—Our society places an emphasis on the superficial trappings of money. I don't feel like I measure up because what I have is not on the same level of what a peer may have. Or, I believe that I should have what I want now and should not have to wait. There is a mentality of deservedness when trying to keep up with the Joneses. The infamous Joneses also have us focusing on the socioeconomic mobility that we can acquire if we make it into their circle. Or maybe the Joneses for you is the guy at the end of the hall in the corner office at your workplace who always seems to get the breaks, the promotions, and the admiration of the rest of the office. I need to be more like him.

At the heart of your struggle is "Am I good enough for someone to value me for me, not for what I have or do?"

Not worthy of goodness—There are many shameful and disgusting instances in far too many people's lives that include the denigration of basic human decency due to molestation, child abuse, or emotional abuse. There can be many things associated with a painful past that cause a person to question whether they are good enough. You may be plagued with shame, guilt, anger, or the inability to forgive. In every instance, the victim is not to blame, should not feel guilty, has the right to be angry and will have to come face to face with forgiveness. The person who robbed you of so much does not determine if you are good enough. Or, maybe you have been hurt by a church that you felt damaged your soul and want to run as far away from people that say they love God as possible as a way to protect yourself. The pain that you experienced may impact your feelings in critical relationships later in life.

The voice in your head may question, "Am I good enough to be loved the way I deserve?"

Not healthy enough—Sometimes life has been hard. It might be an ongoing battle with cancer, a person might be overweight, or might feel like mental illness is just too much to bear. When your body feels like it is physically turning on itself or that it is so far out of control that any little step that you take cannot make a difference, a struggle with not feeling good enough can wreak havoc with your mind. You may feel like giving up or feel like the first step is too big.

Because there is a focus on one ailment, you may not even be able to imagine how to answer a broader question of "Am I good enough to take steps to help myself heal?"

Not a good decision maker—How did you get to the point where your marriage is so horrible that you can't stand the other person's voice? How did the kids get so out of control? There might be many different factors that play into any one of those answers. It might feel like circumstances are beyond your control. But this is where you are. It didn't just happen. Maybe you feel like you never have enough time to become the person that you know you should be. You have created your priorities and are the only one that can change those.

You are in a battle to determine, "Am I good enough to do the hard work that I need to do?"

Being in a constant struggle to try to be good enough is a lost battle. God's unique creation of each one of us answers the question, am I good enough?

Yes, and more!

The amazing thing is that the phrase 'good enough' is truly defined as just meeting a basic requirement when other more rewarding and advanced contentment exists. We cannot get stuck thinking that God only wants to help us see that we are good enough.

He wants so much more for us.

We are trying to be "good enough" rather than working on how to be living in a place of purpose. How He created each of us with unique gifts is where we can revel in His purpose and path.

Do you know what might be keeping you from hearing God's voice? Are you living a life that corresponds to what you believe?

In what areas of your life have you struggled to feel good enough? What will it take for you to move from a place of trying to be good enough to a place of abundant grace?

Take each of the four categories of the trappings of not feeling good enough in this chapter and reread them. This time, at the end of each italicized statement, add the sentence, "God already believes you are. He wants more for you."

Chapter 10

*"The best way to find yourself is to lose
yourself in the service of others."*

—Mahatma Gandhi

Sometimes the battle of seeing the good in yourself is not the easiest place to start. The trappings of our own failings, feelings of inadequacy, and habits of stinking thinking get in the way. The greatest gifts we have are the ones used to support others. In doing so, we help heal ourselves and see how some of our gifts can be used in a way that serves others, not ourselves.

So, start with your gifts. But be careful, the gifts that you have are typically where the "Are we good enough?" doubting begins. It is where we start comparing and doubting our abilities. Do not start with doubt, but rather with your gifts.

A gift is not just the things that we are good at.

Every disability, every blessing, every curse can become gifts for us to live an authentic life. Not a life like everyone else's, but for the purpose God made us for. If God made each of us for a unique purpose, then we should never be comparing. How can your perspective aid others? You have a chance to engage them, not distract them.

At different times in your life, you have different gifts, in the same way that you will have different purposes during different seasons of your life. When I was young, I felt like I had the gift of time. Time didn't really exist until mom yelled that it was time to come in for dinner. Today, time seems to be the gift that I am forever chasing.

The first step is taking stock of your gifts. What are you innately good at? The key is to not think about the "things" that you do, but your connectedness or purpose in doing them. You might say that you are a great carpenter, which might be very true. But is your gift that you work with wood, or is it that you can see the beauty or the potential where others can't? Or, maybe it is that you are a finisher. You have a gift of seeing every project through to the end. Or, maybe you have the ability to see how the creation of a space or environment adds value to other people's lives and can decrease their stress. When you look at your gifts this way, it is not just about a piece of wood.

I have had periods in my life when I did not feel good enough. Reverting to a place of using my gifts helped to ground me and make me feel like I was a positive force. In short, it helped to quiet the voice in my head that was screaming I was not good enough.

It took me a while to figure out my gifts, to move beyond the trappings of comparing myself to others. I have many gifts, but the ones that I am most proud of are my ability to connect and have people understand how they matter to me and my gift of reflection.

But these were not always my gifts.

When I was in college, my roommates would have been very quick to tell you that the first time they met me, they couldn't stand me. They said that I would walk into a room like I was in charge, a little overconfident. But then they got to know me and they loved me for exactly the same reasons. They realized that this was not an act. I really did have a confidence that could be infectious, and I was a bit of a know-it-all. But they also saw that when I was with them, I gave them 100% of my attention—eye contact, asking questions, being completely engaged in what was happening in their lives. They saw how much I cared about their hearts and knew I would do anything for them. I am one of the most loyal people to my friends. I strive to have every interaction with anyone in my life be one where hopefully there is no question as they walk away—I see them and believe that their heart matters. Since my diagnosis, this has been much easier to do.

I have realized the need to put strong words into conversations so that nothing goes unsaid.

After college, when I started my career in education, many people would ask me how I could be a high school history teacher. Didn't the students drive me nuts? Weren't they out of control? No. These raging hormonal teens were my responsibility and every day I was going to reflect on how I could do better, how they could engage more, what practices had to disappear from instruction, how else I could push them, and how I could support their goals. The combination of students feeling like they mattered and this reflection led to a dynamic room full of adventurous learning. Every day was an exercise in reflection. It still is. After starting a non-profit to support breast cancer patients and their families, I am constantly using reflective practices to evaluate and improve our programming and strategic planning.

Identifying and using my gifts was and is a decision that I make, not something that I should wait for others to ask of me. I try to be reflective to hone in on my gifts.

Use this logical deductive questioning and activity to explore the topic and start revealing your own gifts.

Deductive Questioning

What activities and/or tasks do I feel like I am good at or enjoy?

What words describe the feeling that I have when I am engaged in that activity (purposeful, happy, organized, etc.)?

If someone was looking at me through a glass window, what words would they use to describe me?

What would someone else say are your gifts?

Gift Activity

Choose six people (two family members, two friends, one co-worker, one acquaintance) and ask them what they think your gifts are. Be prepared to be quiet and listen. Do not engage in any statements that negate their positive comments.

Write each one down on a piece of paper. Reflect on what they have said and try to look at it from their lens. Have you ever seen yourself like this? Did you like the way that they characterized you? Why or why not?

How can you use the gift that they described to help others?

Chapter 11

When I started treatment or when I have been faced with a family crisis, friends have posed the question, "What can I do to help?" or even worse, "Let me know if you need any help." I have realized that while I was busy trying to figure out how to get through each breath, all of those questions seem too overwhelming to answer because they require energy and effort. There are books out there that will tell people how to come up with specific things to ask of people. Simple tasks, like if they are going to the grocery store, to have them call their friends or family before they go to see if they need anything. During my treatment, I hadn't read those books until after people starting asking, so I didn't know what to ask for.

One of the greatest things I have learned in my lifetime was from people during that time. What I learned was the way in which the people who used their gifts got a chance to grow within their own spirit. I realized that when they used their gifts, they had a chance to say 'I love you' in a way that was meaningful to them, which is what made it even more impactful for me as the receiver.

My sister-in-law Diana is a beautiful example of a person that uses her gifts to bring light into my life. She loves artistic expression through painting. Each week during my treatment, she would listen to the tales of my week and paint a 5x7 canvas that depicted the week, with a quote that summed up my feelings. Every week, I looked forward to seeing how she depicted the horrors and joys of that time. Fifty-four weeks later, I had a huge canvas mural on my wall that tells the story of my cancer journey. She could have chosen to make a casserole or send me flowers. But the choice to use her gift showed me the depth of her love and created a space where she could help heal with her own emotions as she was dealing with her friend and sister's diagnosis.

When I started treatment, I had the ugliest bathroom on the planet. Imagine an avocado green bathtub, a tiffany blue sink, a harvest gold toilet and blue floral wallpaper with geese who—if they had a choice over the years—probably would have flown off the wall, just to get away from the clashing colors. It was the worst place imaginable to start my day. My brothers and sisters decided that if there was a possibility that the treatment would cause me to get sick, they wanted me to at least have a bathroom that wasn't completely hideous and nauseating in its own right. They chose to completely remodel my bathroom in one day. Two days before my first chemo, they convinced my husband to take me away, and I returned to a complete surprise at the end of the day. The bathroom definitely looked better. But the wallpaper glue shows through and the bathroom tub white epoxy didn't quite cover all of the avocado splendor in the shower. But their gift wasn't the finished bathroom at all. It was one of the gifts that mattered the most to me—the gift of strength and family unity. There was no way my five brothers and sisters were going to ever give me a chance to feel like I was alone, even though all of us were in different parts of the country.

I had set a goal at the beginning of treatment that I would continue to walk each and every day. Cancer would not take that away from me. I had a dear friend, Melissa, who made it a priority to make sure that every single day I walked a mile. She met me at the track, she picked me up, she created ways to continue to keep me going even when I did not want to go. She never focused on my cancer, but rather always on getting me stronger. Every time she talked about how I was getting stronger, even though I felt like I was getting weaker and weaker, I would see the hope of being done with treatment. The hope that I would be able to take a walk without feeling horrible. Her constant positive attitude and encouraging words were her gifts that she used to serve me during a horrible time. There was no casserole that could ever compare to the gift of her friendship.

These people were ridiculously present in my life. They showed up when it mattered. That was their gift. That is the gift that all of us have to give.

When we start using our gifts, our true gifts, we get the opportunity to become ridiculously present for others, and in turn, start to live a more authentic life.

We become the least important person in the equation.

We start listening.

We start having the ability to see God in the small, in-between spaces of our life.

We start having the ability to see a nudge as a nudge and not a coincidence.

We start feeling self-worth, not because of what we are doing, but because of how we are living in a space with our best self.

What are my gifts?

How am I using the gifts that I have to serve others?

Chapter 12

The idea behind the nonprofit Little Pink Houses of Hope is actually pretty simple. There are empty rental vacation properties all over the country. If I could just find a way to coordinate the empty ones so that they were donated the same week, I could then work on creating a schedule to help support families have the most amazing week of their lives. The problem was that I had the idea, but didn't know exactly what to do with it. So I started googling. To this day, I am convinced that Google can do wonders to help people take God's little nudges and make them into a reality.

After starting Little Pink Houses of Hope, I was completely unsure how a business model for people to donate their homes and secure donated meals and services would ever work. I had the idea clearly in my head, but would people actually agree when I asked them to be a part of the program? What I found was that the same affirmation that my sister, my siblings, my friend, and countless others along the way gave when given a chance to find themselves using their gifts for others. The most profound thing that I learned was that there were people just like me who had been getting nudges and ignoring them that would love the chance to say YES!

The very first person that I ever asked for anything of was a wild woman in a pink pancake house. I was scouting out our first retreat location in Carolina Beach, NC. I was driving down the main road and was drawn to her restaurant. You cannot miss the dedication of her restaurant to the color pink! At this point, I was grasping for any sign, so a restaurant painted pink partnering with an organization that served breast cancer families seemed like a logical choice.

I had said yes to God, but now I had to make it happen.

I walked into the restaurant and asked to speak to the owner, Kate. I was standing in front of this magnanimous, smiling woman, who said, "I'm her sweetie, what's up?" Tripping over my tongue, I strung together words about what I was trying to do.

"I want to create a place for cancer patients to come and get away for a week."

"It will be for families getting a break from their cancer."

"Could you maybe, please, donate a breakfast for some of the families?"

Even though the organizational elevator speech was not rehearsed or probably even very coherent, without hesitation, she threw her hands up in the air and said YES!

I couldn't believe it. Not only had she said yes, but she seemed excited about something she barely knew anything about. In that moment, God had clearly put her in my path. Still to this day, that yes was the most important one that has ever happened because it caused me to see very clearly the power of the organization that I created. I have the privilege of watching people's lives unfold to become involved in directly serving others. I have a front row seat at how God moves and works through people.

I realized that I had always had a front row seat, but I was just not ridiculously present enough to be able to realize it until now.

Little did I know that Kate was waiting for me to walk in. Her backstory was that she had been searching for a purpose that was bigger than herself. She knew that she was being pulled for something more, a way to give back to her community. I didn't know that she had been having her own nudges, but I had been lucky enough to walk in and give her the final push! Caring for people through food was one of the gifts that her grandmother had instilled so deeply into her. Over the years, Kate has gone from donating a meal, to planning an entire retreat, to raising over $50,000 for our organization, using every one of her gifts to directly serve families in need. And it all started with her saying yes to using her gifts. She will be the first person to tell you that in a lifetime full of trying to make good decisions and questioning whether she was good enough for x, y, or z throughout her life, her decision to say yes has been a decision where God clearly exists and holds her in the palm of His hand.

Using the gifts that God has given us is about making the decision to say YES! Some people are looking to have others walk right in and ask them to use their gifts, and may wait a lifetime. Imagine if all of the gifts that God carefully crafted into you were never shared with the world. Imagine if your gift is necessary for someone else's gift to be fully realized. I have often thought that God has uniquely made all of us, but that we are all part of a much larger tapestry. There is an interconnectedness in all of us that requires us to find the ability to use our gifts to serve others and be ridiculously present in the lives of people around us.

What fears and insecurities do I need to get rid of to be able to say YES when God walks in and asks me to use my gift to do His work?

Chapter 13

I have always been a type A fixer. I want to help. I want to solve. I want to make someone else's pain go away. I want to be able to have their life be better because of my help. But when I got cancer, I realized that sometimes there is no fix. And the people who touched me the most weren't the people with the answers, but the people who knew how to serve, rather than help. It became clear to me that when people served, I learned to be more ridiculously present in that relationship. Their service somehow got through to me in a way that nothing else had. Their service allowed me to see my own goodness in a life where I had not been able to see God for a long time.

Identifying the gifts that we can share and then saying yes are two of the first steps we need to take when we feel lost or can't see God. It creates an environment of openness, and when individuals use their gifts to serve, it sets the stage to be ridiculously present. Being ridiculously present is not about fixing you or what I can get from you, but rather seeing your wholeness and walking alongside you.

My mom is a wonderful example of a faith-filled woman with a servant's heart. My older sister, Kristie, had attended a summer camp when she was a teenager and my mother sent her an article, since she was on the precipice of being on her own and figuring out her own faith and what she believed. Years later, as I was putting together the programming for the first year of Little Pink, my sister shared the article with me, and I have passed it on to friends. For years, every volunteer that serves our families on a Little Pink Houses of Hope weeklong breast cancer retreat, has read the article by Rachel Ramen, *In the Service of Life*. The article beautifully explains the difference between helping, fixing, and serving. This difference is at the heart of the definition of being ridiculously present. Ramen explains:

> Serving is different from helping. Helping is based on inequality; it is not a relationship between equals. When you help, you use your own strength to help those of lesser strength ... If I'm attentive to what's going on inside of me when I'm helping, I find that I'm always helping someone who's not as strong as I am, who is needier than I am.

> When I help I am very aware of my own strength. But we don't serve with our strength, we serve with ourselves ... Our limitations serve, our wounds serve, even our darkness can serve. The wholeness in us serves the wholeness in others and the wholeness in life. The wholeness in you is the same as the wholeness in me. Service is a relationship between equals ...

> When I fix a person, I perceive them as broken, and their brokenness requires me to act. When I fix, I do not see the wholeness in the other person or trust the integrity of the life in them. When I serve, I see and trust that wholeness.

> Helping incurs debt. When you help someone, they owe you one. But serving, like healing, is mutual. There is no debt. I am as served as the person I am serving. When I help I have a feeling of satisfaction. When I serve I have a feeling of gratitude …

At the heart of service is the desire to aid in letting another person's heart breathe; to create space for the wonder of the day to be something that can be marveled at; to walk alongside someone who is burdened in a way that the load is shared and doesn't feel quite so heavy.

I am guilty of trying to "fix" people in my life, and it always starts from a place of judgment.

If only she would do this …

Can't he see that this is the right decision …

If they would just stop doing that …

Living in a place of judgment of others is a dangerous place to live because it is rooted in the belief that others are not as good as you perceive yourself. How can you be a positive part of their life if you can't even see them?

To understand judgment better, imagine that there is a brick wall between you and the person being judged. A wall has been erected to separate you from their failings. But you still think that you can see everything through the brick wall, and you are sure that your side of the wall is better than theirs. We are willing to do what we want to have the other person move to our side of the wall, but rarely are we willing to leave our judgment on our side of the wall and stand beside them in their place of brokenness. We want to fix the problem, but are not willing to sit with them as they go through their pain.

It is impossible to be ridiculously present when we are busy comparing ourselves and basking in any feelings of superiority. The only way to serve others is to eliminate the idea of fixing the other person and decide that serving alongside them is what we have to offer.

We cannot be ridiculously present with others if we stay on our side of the brick wall.

This journey has made me realize that I have put up a brick wall with God and other people. Any feelings of unworthiness or shame caused me to erect a wall, making the judgement of others easy and closing me off from letting Him walk alongside me in my brokenness.

Do you have people that you have tried to "fix"?

How would that situation have turned out if you had seen their wholeness and walked alongside them, rather than trying to "fix" them?

Do you have a wall up against God?

Chapter 14

My cancer treatment gave me a unique opportunity to experience people walking alongside me using their gifts.

I didn't know what to expect with my first chemotherapy treatment, except that my regimen would last a total of eight to nine hours every third week. I made the decision that I did not want to burden any one particular person with my treatment schedule, but rather that I would have a different person attend each treatment with me. I was very selfishly looking forward to the time that I had with each person. I worried that with a grave diagnosis, if I didn't make it, I would make the most of the quality time with the people that I love on each treatment day.

My sister-in-law Diana drew the lucky straw for being my chemo buddy for the first treatment. I could not have picked a better person for the first day. Diana is a cornucopia of arts and crafts fun on a normal day, but she took her chemo assignment seriously. We were going to have fun! Diana came loaded with four bags of magazines, blankets, pillows, food, tea, DVDs, and a gift bag containing letters from people on Team Jeanine. My mom had the brainchild to reach out to various people in my life to write letters for me to open on my first day of chemo. It was an amazing idea. Reading through all of the cards and notes helped surround me with the people who cared and loved me the most.

Diana made sure that there was not a single moment for me to think about the toxic liquids pouring into my body.

She had created the best girl's day ever.

As we were walking out of the chemo room, we stopped at the nurse's station and I remember saying, "I love chemo day!" You could see from the looks on the nurses' faces that they knew more than I did about what was coming. But Diana had created an environment that made sure that if it was going to get worse from here, we might as well celebrate the days that didn't seem so bad.

She was all in. She was ridiculously present, attending to my soul that day.

There was no agenda of fixing my cancer, or how she was going to change that she couldn't help me. She could, however, be in a place of service to my soul and give the gift of joy and optimism.

My brother Jason was the winner of the chemo day lottery for my second treatment. My hair had fallen out, but I still felt like I could handle anything, until my world flipped upside down. They had warned me during my first round of chemo of the side effects. Red face, stabbing back pain, inability to breathe, possible heart issues—you know, the typical run-of-the-mill toxic poison kind of stuff. Nothing had happened during the first chemo, so I was not worried. About forty-five minutes into treatment, I looked at Jason and said "Go get help." I am glad that I got that out before my breathing dropped to nothing, my face turned as red as a Coke can, my heart rate soared and five people rushed into the room to hook me up to machines and administer more medicine than I could imagine. It was incredibly scary, to say the least.

And through it all, my little brother was Mr. Cool under pressure. He had a calmness about him and his words of reassurance were constant. He was not trying to convince himself that it would be OK. Rather, he was completely in charge and was only making sure that I knew I would be fine. I had always thought of him as my silly little brother. Sharing his gift of protection and compassion that day caused me to see him for the first time. He is stronger than I ever imagined, or more fitting, than I ever realized. Jason had given me a wonderful lesson in how to let others care for and protect me.

I did not always have to be the strongest person in the room.

When I spoke with my sister later that weekend and recounted the story of my treatment day, she said that my cancer was a chance to "let the rest of us find our way to be better people and show you our greatness though all of this."

I thought about that very intently. Our burdens and our brokenness can seem overwhelming to us, but they offer opportunities for others to become ridiculously present in our lives, if we let them. Not only do we have to answer the call to walk alongside others, we have a duty to let others be a part of our journey and prop us up.

Little did I know that my third chemo treatment would be one of the best gifts I could receive. My mom had come, ready to be a mom and take care of me. Her baby girl was struggling and was physically exhausted. I had different plans. I had come up with a list of 10 questions for us to answer. The day was filled with stories of her life, the details of her lifelong love affair with my dad and what her dreams and goals had been. She became exactly who I needed her to be that day. At the end of the day, we were both oddly sad when we had to leave the chemotherapy suite. With my dad dying 15 months later, the stories that I heard were one of the most precious gifts that I could imagine her sharing.

The next twelve months of treatment all followed suit. Each included a person who was close to me making the decision to be ridiculously present in my life for the day. Each gift of their love that they brought left an indelible mark on my soul. They were not going to fix anything or help my cancer disappear, but they could be ridiculously present and walk alongside me on the journey.

There was no way that they were going to just "go through the motions."

So, if when we think someone might be dying, we refuse to settle on just going through the motions, how is it that we struggle to make the same decision with the rest of our days?

When is the last time you were ridiculously present with another person?

What keeps you from doing this more?

When others have tried to be ridiculously present in your life, have you let them have the opportunity to do so?

Chapter 15

The goal of becoming authentic is to go from a place of worrying about being good enough to loving who you are, even in your brokenness.

Being authentic is hard.

I have found that it is the only space in which I can now live. Being less than authentic feels like I am wasting my time, whatever amount I have left, on superficial nonsense. The goal of being authentic is looking at who you really are, what you truly believe, loving your faults and imperfections and realizing that they create your unique ability to grow and change. Not running from them—but really seeing them. And cherishing all of your good qualities. Celebrating what makes you unique without apology, but being humble enough to know that internally celebrating your gifts can give you more strength than imaginable. Understanding when you don't feel good enough that you are not loving yourself and that is not okay.

Making the decision to be authentic was about being true to my heart and soul—but it required me to really look at what I believed to be able to get there. It required difficult decisions and prioritizing all aspects of my life. It required saying no when I didn't want to and yes when I didn't want to.

To do this, you must let yourself be vulnerable, which is one of the hardest things EVER. Vulnerability is not about being weak, but rather having a strength to let others in to walk alongside you. Accepting God's purpose in your life is also the process of becoming totally vulnerable to a God that loves you.

A year after starting the breast cancer nonprofit, Little Pink Houses of Hope, I was working at least 80 hours a week out of my living-room-turned-office on the planning and coordination of our programming and feeling the weight of the world on my shoulders. There were so many families applying for retreats. How could we ever serve them all? I continued to work at my education-training job, traveling around the state at least 60 hours per week.

What in the world was I thinking?

In an attempt to help other people and answer God's calling, I was undoubtedly headed on a path that was going to make me sick again. My husband was worried beyond belief. I was giving all of myself away to others and he could sense that I was feeling conflicted about the choice I made. Not because it was the wrong choice, but because it was a hard choice that had financial implications for my family.

I was faced with the question, "How do you act on a big calling when the mortgage needs to be paid and you need insurance?"

We were back at the beach, three years after the initial calling. Same house. Same beach. But everything was different at this point. I had thought that I had answered God's calling. I had started Little Pink Houses of Hope, which had become a great model for breast cancer family support. But I had no idea how I could keep going. I was tired. Not because of the cancer, but because I was struggling to understand how to continue the dual role with my job and my newfound passion, Little Pink Houses of Hope.

So, I went for a run. The same path that I ran on the day that He had called me to serve Him. Only this time, as I approached the gates to the compound that had changed my life years before, they were open. The compound had recently been purchased and was in the initial stages of being remodeled. There was lots of work to do. Years of neglect, ocean weathering, and being uninhabited created structural issues. But it was exciting to see the possibility of how it might be able to come back to life. As I was running through the compound, the overwhelming push and pull tension of my life weighed very heavy. I started crying, not able to answer the question, "How can I keep doing both of these jobs?" By this point, it was clear that I had answered His initial call, but how do I remain obedient and still be able to provide for my family? I had run to the back of the compound and was turning around to run back when that same voice of my soul became crystal clear.

> *I have taken care of you. Trust me.*
> *I have taken care of you. Trust me.*

For whatever reason, God comes to me and always says things twice, which is a good thing, because I am clearly a slow learner. Again, the same physical reaction. I felt completely clear in my mind and His love was reverberating in my heart. He had struck again. I took a couple more steps and then started immediately with the stinking thinking.

"You want me to trust you, but haven't I already trusted you?"

"You clearly have taken care of seeding and growing Little Pink Houses of Hope, but how can I take care of my family?"

"How can I be obedient to your will without causing a burden on my family?"

What I was really asking was, how can I take a real leap of faith with Him?

I continued to run to the compound exit and came across a man in a ditch, working. I stopped, just to thank him for helping to restore the place so that others would be able to enjoy it. He reached his hand out and said, "Hi! My name is Jim. I am the new owner." I proceeded to tell Jim all about the original run around his compound, the calling, and the subsequent creation of Little Pink Houses of Hope. He told me all about his history with the Navy, why he purchased the property, and his plans for its future. At the end of the conversation, he told me that when he got them all fixed up, he would let me use them for one of my retreats. "You have a strong faith in God, so I will give you a week and we will have to see if this God guy you talk about shows up." I could feel God just giggling at me. You want a sign, here you go.

I knew in that moment that what was holding me back from fully committing to God's calling was that I had been looking at it as needing to take a leap of faith and that seemed way too difficult. Would He be there to catch me? What if I didn't have what it takes to be successful? What if at my core I was just a shallow person who didn't want to do without the material things to which I had become accustomed? What if I wasn't good enough?

And then it hit me.

God asked me, not anybody else to do this one thing. He asked me to change my life and give it over to Him. I could say that I believed, but did I really believe in His ability to make ANYTHING happen? I had seen evidence in every interaction while building Little Pink. Numerous business owners, community members, and individuals all shared their stories of the opportunity to be a part of God's work and give back. I had seen evidence of the way in which I had interactions with people that He clearly put on my path. What other evidence did I need?

And that was when I realized that He was not asking for a leap of faith.

It was a leap of assurance.

He had given me instruction in the first calling to create a place for people to come. In the second calling, He had reassured me that He would care for me if I trusted Him. A leap of faith would have been hoping that I was making the right decision and hoping that He would be there. No, when God calls you, pushes you, nudges you, He is asking you to take a leap of assurance. He will be there to catch you. He will walk alongside you each and every step of the way. The steps may be hard and seem like a rocky path, but He is with you. It is a leap of assurance.

I went from being at my wit's end to returning to the beach house with a plan. I wrote my entire plan down in my journal. I would quit my job by this date. I would get medical insurance through this process. I would lean into the opportunities to simplify our lives and rely on others for help.

I am not saying, quit your job today without a plan. I am saying to think about how the decision affects you and everyone that matters, and come up with a plan. If it is about quitting your job, you will have to take a serious look at the money you'll need.

This was one of the first lessons my husband and I learned about the way in which God had placed people in our path to help us on our journey, long before this calling. Our son, Jake, went to a private school from kindergarten through 8th grade. We could not imagine him going anywhere else for high school. Academic success was important to us and deep down I was worried that if my cancer came back, I would need to ensure he would be surrounded by people that knew him and loved our family. I prayed one night about how to be obedient and forego my salary without forcing Jake into public school. What seemed like a trade-off that would be detrimental to our son turned into a necessary lesson in humility.

When God calls you to do one thing, it comes with all of these other lessons along the way.

I scheduled a meeting with the principal of the school and told him that we were struggling. We knew that I needed to quit my job and continue the path laid out for me, but it would be at the expense of our son's education. We felt like God was calling us to march forward with Little Pink but also to keep Jake at his school. We told them that we needed help. Without missing a beat, the principal said, let us care for your family. God has trusted you with this mission, let us be a part of that trust. He had almost reiterated the same words that God had used. They immediately reduced Jake's tuition, removing that burden from our lives. God had placed this loving community in our lives for years and it took a humbling experience for us to see that His promise on that second run, "I will take care of you, if you trust me," wasn't just small talk.

Going to Jake's school was not a difficult decision, but a humbling one.

God put the loving people of his school in our path years prior to our meeting. It is a disservice not to use them. I needed to learn the art of receiving. You don't have to have something to give to someone when they bestow a gift upon you. When someone gives you something, you can rob them of their chance to be a blessing by making it a transaction.

How much do you trust that God will care for you?

Have you ever thought that there was no way out of a difficult situation because you were only looking at options that were easy, or options that did not require sacrifice?

Can you abandon the trappings of this life to do the will of God?

Chapter 16

The hard choice lies in listening to your purpose and God's calling and then breathing life into your actions. Being ridiculously present is not enough if you are not ridiculously active. What you do is THE thing that matters. It takes planning, but it also takes believing that it is not a leap of faith, but a leap of assurance. Plan it out and look at all of the pieces of the puzzle.

So many times, I had to realize that I was still operating on my version of how the puzzle fits together. God might have only shown me one quarter of the puzzle of the picture that I was creating. That partially completed puzzle to me might look different than the whole picture, and might definitely be different than what God had planned. Planning my life around being ridiculously present with God was different than sticking to my plan.

Being ridiculously present requires a flexibility that is unimaginable.

Going from a place of wondering about your worth to purposeful living with God often requires reckless abandon.

When people hear the phrase 'reckless abandon,' they often times think of a rowdy, out-of-control party. Mine is a story of reckless abandon. God has created this amazing party with guests that I did not know, loud music, and disruptive chaos. To enter into the party, I had to decide to leave my ego at the door. To be open to His calling, God needed me to put my academic elitism in the coat check area. I had to surrender my diagnosis and accept that I might not make it out alive. I had to talk to complete strangers and learn how to dance completely differently.

It was the most chaotic party that I have ever attended, because it was the party God had designed to celebrate my gifts.

God creates these parties to let individuals know that they are the most important guest—because they are His.

More importantly, He wants for us to leave the party and never go to another party the same way ever again. I had a choice to abandon the financial and emotional comfort that I knew and become ridiculously present with God.

The idea was unimaginable at first. I had barely wanted to listen to God's calling, so the decision to become ridiculously present with Him was a foreign concept. It was at this point that the questions of whether I was good enough started creeping to the surface again. Could I be all in? What if I had to make choices and decisions that caused me to lose everything? What if this next step was the one where my family decided enough is enough? And therein lies another major aspect of accepting God's purpose for your life.

The people that we love are often in completely different places of their life spiritually, emotionally, and in terms of readiness.

How do we balance what our heart is telling us we should do with what the people that we love still need from us? It is in that space where relationships grow. This can be a very difficult space, full of conflict, arguments, and pain. This aspect of the journey can take over as the disruptive chaos that can be experienced at God's party of reckless abandon.

The decision to quit my job, forego health insurance, lose my salary, and dedicate my life to helping others was our greatest marital strain. We were in two different places spiritually. At the core of our issue was that my husband remains worried every single day that my cancer will return. And rightfully so, he is entitled to have this fear and I must learn to respect that he does not want anything to happen to the woman that he loves. He dedicated his life to me, not this calling. There were numerous conversations that all looked similar:

Me: I know that God will take care of it.

Him: Tell me how God is going to pay our bills.

Me: I can't keep doing two jobs.

Him: Exactly, but which one pays the bills? I get that you can't walk away from Little Pink, but we still have to pay our bills.

Me: I trust that He will take care of it.

Over and over again, we had this conversation.

I had this newfound relationship with God that intimidated him somewhat. In all honesty, he probably felt somewhat left out, since he was not part of the discussions with God. Throughout this journey, my husband has moved at a different speed of acceptance than me, which is to be expected. His running joke is that he understands that God is talking to me and calling me to change our lives, but just once, he would like God to just give him a sticky note of what is coming up.

Just a sticky note.

Our conversations slowly turned from not understanding how it could work to exploring what would happen if I moved to part time, then quarter time, eventually getting to the point where quitting altogether seemed possible. I look back at this time and realize one very important lesson that is not to be missed. As a couple, we worked through this together. I could have completely railroaded him into doing it my way. I could have walked in and quit and told him that that was how it was going to be. But that would not have been part of God's plans for our vows. It would not have respected the love and care that we need to show to each other. Those six months were very hard, but we grew tremendously as a couple because we became ridiculously present with each other. We listened, compromised, and in the end, it was our choice—not mine.

God was calling my entire family to do this, but was only speaking to me.

I have never felt lighter than on the day I turned in my resignation. The weight and burden was lifted. I no longer worried about how to make it work without insurance and a salary. I reveled in the opportunity to watch how God would care for us. I had just recently established a brand new board of directors at Little Pink Houses of Hope and they were going through their own training process. I would come home and my husband would ask, "Can't you just give yourself a salary?" No, it was something that the board would need to decide, and they have work to do to get to that point. I went from being the major breadwinner in our home to going without a salary for five months. We had depleted our savings during my cancer treatment with copays, out of pocket expenses, and treatments that were not covered. We made the decision to use some of my retirement money to take the financial pressure off of us.

We survived.

The decision to be ridiculously present with God was about accepting that He has created a space where a leap of assurance is mandatory. It is the cost of admittance to His party of reckless abandon.

Are you ready to get an invite to God's party?

What would a life of reckless abandon look like in your life?

Are there relationships in your life that seem like they are holding you back from answering God's call? How can you become ridiculously present with that person to move forward?

What would happen to your life if you started living a life that God had imagined for you? Would you be richer or poorer, and how?

Chapter 17

You cannot be ridiculously present unless you go out into the world with your gifts, live your vulnerability, and be the hands and feet of God. If you are only ever present with your own thoughts, you are actually not living an authentic life.

The most rewarding, amazing, and fulfilling time of your life can come when you are ridiculously present, hear God's voice and act upon His path for your life.

But that doesn't mean that it might not totally suck.

The reality of being ridiculously present doesn't just mean for the good stuff. You will witness the heartache and pain of the death of the person that you are closest to or a child that commits suicide. When you break down your walls of judgment and walk alongside people in pain, your heart will break. When disruptive chaos is coming at you, you will want to give up. Being ridiculously present requires levels of emotional engagement that most people don't typically experience. You may have to sacrifice, you may question yourself, you may even question why God would lead you into the lion's den, but you must go through this aspect of being ridiculously present.

It is where you will find His face, your strength, and your ability to see His abundant grace for your life.

Engaging means you also have to deal with what others may think of you. Others may attack you, call you foolish, question your motives, or try to put up roadblocks to help meet their emotional needs. You will have to be reflective of other's motives and separate them from your own.

There have been many instrumental people in my life in creating Little Pink, each with a special gift that God placed in my path to help me along this journey. They have given me strength, shown love, and cared for my soul. One such volunteer had found her purpose through helping our families, and it was a beautiful vehicle for God's gifts to shine. The reality, though, was that it caused a rift in her marriage. The travel, the focus outside the family, and the changing roles of the family that her volunteering left was her disruptive chaos. It was a difficult time and I encouraged her to have her family attend a retreat as volunteers so that they could witness the work that she was doing and experience firsthand how God was shining through her.

Every year, June 15 is my cancerversary, a day commemorating my diagnosis. It is a day full of mixed emotions. There is a sense of time that has passed where "you have made it" and a sense of the possibility of being closer to being re-diagnosed. In the first year of our retreats, that day fell during a retreat week, the week that I had invited her family to attend. I woke up and went for a walk on the beach. I had a long talk with God that morning that was full of gratitude for all of the wonderful things that He had done in caring for me.

I thanked Him for showing up in my life and pursuing me.

As I returned from my walk and was walking up the boardwalk stairs, I found my friend that was very close to me, who was pivotal in helping to implement the Little Pink retreat programming, sitting on the steps. She was on the steps with her husband and I could tell she had been crying.

Her husband approached me in a fit of rage. I was the punching bag that he unleashed his verbal attack at, without holding anything back. The attack on my personal character, the work that we were doing, the way in which he felt this work was tearing his marriage apart were coming at me at warp speed. I stood there with a calmness that is hard to explain. I could feel God shielding me. With my friend curled up in a ball on the step, I realized that this attack was less about me and more about issues within their own marriage. I could fight back or I could let his venom spew and be there to care for my friend when it was done. I chose the latter. It was a vicious attack, which stuck with me for a very long time. I do not have a history of physical or verbal abuse in my past, so to have someone screaming insults at me and physically coming into my space to intimidate me was something that frightened and terrorized me.

He was looking for me to kick him out and tell him to go home. He was looking for me to be the reason that his wife would have to quit. He was looking to control an out-of-control situation in his world.

He had vehemently told me that I was not good enough— not good enough to be the organizational leader, to be his wife's friend, to care for cancer patients and that I was not making a difference in the world. For the first time in a long time, the self-doubt did not creep in. It is when we are caught up in the worldly comparisons or the doubt of our own self-worth or purpose that feelings of inadequacy seep in. As he said these words, I realized that I do not need him to think that I am good enough.

God believes that I am so much more.

I spent the next few months in full support of her, listening to the decisions that she was facing. I was ridiculously present in a situation where it was incredibly difficult to separate my own feelings from hers.

But I showed up and I was ridiculously present—even though it broke my heart.

During that time, it became clear how the aggressive nature of the situation that day on the beach was rooted in someone that needed his pain to become mine.

The situation with my friend was difficult. We were moving at different speeds of forgiveness with the issues with her husband. She was used to forgiving her husband with each new apology.

I needed that extra time to jump into God's arms and rest. She needed me to move at a different speed. Looking back on the experience now, it is easy to see how the energy that I was putting into "fixing" this situation was keeping me from focusing on God's purpose. I couldn't figure out how to come from a place of service because I was hurt. I was incapable of doing it at her speed and ultimately our friendship fell apart.

The lesson I learned was that God puts various people in our lives for various periods of time. My friend and I were together for a period that was necessary for us to see important gifts in our lives, grow in our faith, and learn to be ridiculously present in the lives of others. She had used her gifts and I had been a witness to them. I learned and grew from her. But I continued to move on. I did not let the destructive chaos of her situation keep me from continuing on the path that God had set into motion.

It was when this sort of attack happened that I realized it was most important for me to decide to be ridiculously present with God and His plans. I was faced with the decision to change my circle of influence, reevaluate my long term commitment to our friendship, and take time for forgiveness and healing. In that in-between space, it was so important that I had to remember not to close my eyes to up above on a daily basis.

It is in these in-between spaces that God showed up to carry me.

I had to be humble and let Him in. I did not have to be strong for Him to carry me. I did not have to be weak. The only thing that I had to do was jump into His arms and rest for a little while.

But that didn't mean that I should choose not to be ridiculously present. I have found that sometimes we need to be ridiculously present with the grief and pain that we experience. It is when we avoid being present that our hearts start creeping in with the question, "Am I good enough?"

When things go wrong, is that when it seems like you cannot hear God's voice?

When is the last time that you were able to have adversity in your life and still see God's hand or purpose?

Chapter 18

Making a decision to be ridiculously present with others and with God is a decision. It is a decision that requires other decisions in your life to be made to clear out the noise and trappings of this life. Little Pink has continued to grow into a national nonprofit that provides an amazing opportunity for families to feel God's love on their difficult cancer journey. Each week is an opportunity for families and volunstars (that's what we call our volunteers) to be ridiculously present in each other's lives.

The organization provides a beautiful home, all of the meals, activities, and services for the families at no cost. There are typically 11 families that attend a retreat week and we offer 16 to 20 retreats per year in various locations around the country. Consistently, Little Pink Houses of Hope provides families a chance to hit the pause button on the exhausting treatments, doctor appointments, and daily schedules. This pause button is an important aspect in finding a way to be ridiculously present for others.

Standing in the way for most people in making the decision to be ridiculously present is a litany of excuses that include:

"I don't have enough time."

"I am too busy."

"All of my time is used up caring for my family."

"I don't have money to give to others."

But they are just excuses. If we take a Little Pink Houses of Hope retreat week and dissect it so that we can apply lessons in our own lives as to how to become ridiculously present, we can build a roadmap for our own lives.

Each family is assigned to a house for their retreat week. They do not know anything about the house prior to their arrival.

Families are accepted into a specific retreat week, make travel reservations, arrange for their kids to be out of school, take time off of work and have no idea if there will be anything on the other end when they arrive. They are not given a home address, rather a check in location, usually a church or community center. In a world driven by googling everything, they are not given a link to the home or any additional information. This is the first piece of creating an environment of being ridiculously present. We purposefully remove all expectations. When families show up, they often look like a deer in the headlights. They don't know what to expect. They are greeted by a volunstar who already knows their names and is 100% dedicated to their joyfulness and support for the week.

Imagine going to work today without an expectation that a certain person was going to drive you nuts. Or, if your day is full of car pool tasks, imagine realizing that your kids expect you to pick them up, but you have the ability to have no expectation of the joy that can fill the car. The expectations that we place on our daily activities and interactions impact our abilities to truly see people. We have created a judgment or a wall of expectation that often does not allow us to be present enough to walk alongside another person that we come in contact with.

Families arrive not knowing anything about the schedule for the week. They are given this information at the initial first night dinner. There is no schedule online ahead of time.

Families arrive in a place of wonder. We create a week of the best of the best in each retreat community. We reach out to local community restaurants and vendors for activities and meals.

Many activities on a Little Pink schedule are things that families have never tried before. With little time to think about how they can talk themselves out of an experience, families expand their horizons and explore new aspects of themselves.

So immediately, reading that last paragraph, I am sure that your task list for the week started creeping in. Or, maybe you thought of how if you had someone to prepare your meals, that you too would have more time to be present in the lives of the people that matter. I get it! But, imagine how much richer your life could be if you would say yes to some new experiences. Imagine that you have a gift that God wants you to explore in a new environment. We become people of incredible routines to get through our busy on-demand days.

Activities like playing on the beach, eating out, and riding bikes are all common experiences on all of our retreats. But on our retreat weeks, they take on new meaning. Imagine that you look at your current experiences with a new joy. The activity becomes a time to be ridiculously present with your family, not another task on the list. This tiny little shift is a first step.

Every activity and meal is optional, except the initial and closing meeting. Even though everything is optional, families attend almost all experiences.

The comment that we hear over and over again is that families love the retreat week because people with similar life circumstances surround them. Their children want to play with the other children that are on the retreat. Kids have no worries that their parent is the only one with cancer. Our retreats help to normalize the cancer experience for every family member. Over and over again, I have seen women check in with their wig on the first day. After meeting everyone, they feel liberated to ditch the wig and be free of the trappings of fitting in. As with any crisis, it is exhausting to put on a strong face and spend exhaustive energy making other people feel better. Similarity is important. Not isolation from others, but the addition of a similar tribe.

Imagine if in your own life you chose to surround yourself with others going through similar experiences. Maybe you are grieving the loss of a parent. Part of being ridiculously present in that experience is being able to express your emotions with others going though the same experience. Or, maybe you are a new mom that is struggling with the demands of parenting. Reach out to a Mommy and Me group so that you eliminate the sense of feeling alone every day. There is a schedule that you have to follow and a schedule that you get to create. There are ways to clear up time in your life for things that you prioritize. You may have to get up half an hour earlier to work out and give yourself the time that you need. You may find yourself having to say no to unimportant tasks. You may have to give up your goal of being the "perfect mom" so that your children can see that they matter more than the tasks in your life. But becoming ridiculously present is also rooted in caring for yourself.

Every morning at the volunstar house, the day starts with a meeting to help center the group.

Some retreat directors use inspirational quotes, others incorporate devotions, some play music, but all of these meetings have one thing in common—the day starts with intentionality.

Start every day with some routine of intentionality. Prioritizing this and reminding yourself throughout the day of your purpose will provide you with clarity of mind in a rushed world. Being intentional with your time is key to becoming ridiculously present. If I start the day with the intention of loving everyone that crosses my path, it forces me to give more to every interaction during the day. It causes me to not see these moments as interferences in my day, but opportunities to explore the people that God has placed in my path today and to see God in their faces.

Every night at the volunstar house, the Retreat director leads a meeting with the topic, "What is the best part of your day?"

Invariably, funny stories of the day, emotional connections made, and touching moments dominate the conversation. It is often difficult for volunstars to limit their answer to just one thing. The day is intentional because of how we started it together. The day ends in a place of gratitude. Keep in mind, many days we can have a plethora of things that have gone wrong. Winds that blow the beach tent away, a bee sting, a child that is driving everyone nuts, a breast cancer participant that struggles to walk up a flight of stairs, two teenage kids trying desperately to sneak off together and create their own fun. The list goes on and on. But the end of the day meeting is always rooted in gratitude. And what I have seen is that it is the small tender moments that people recognize and are able to refer back to their own lives that make the greatest impact. Volunstars make a seven-day, 24-hour-a-day commitment during a retreat week. They live together, sleep together and make the week a success by their interactions. They are a family.

Imagine if every single day, your family was intentional about being grateful for people and experiences throughout the day. What I notice as the week progresses is that volunstars will come up to me at midday and say, "I already had the best part of my day." In this environment of intentionality, individuals start looking for their grateful moments and appreciating them throughout the day. Sharing them is just the way in which we can connect the meaning of our day with the people that we love.

Throughout the retreat week, volunstars provide support for the families, both physically and emotionally.

It might be playing with a kid in the sand while her mother talks to another breast cancer survivor, or it might be setting up beach chairs and a tent so that families can arrive and not have to worry about anything. The way in which the volunstars help is immeasurable. But at the core of this aspect of volunteering is being ridiculously present enough to anticipate the needs of others. How often are we so consumed with our own needs that it is too difficult to see how we can serve someone else? Think about your marriage: how could you help serve your spouse so that they could have a better day? We spend plenty of time yelling at our children, but how might you serve them today? That may seem like a crazy notion, because as a parent, it seems like we are always serving them, but how can we get them to see how to care for others while caring for ourselves?

My son has been doing his laundry since the sixth grade, shortly after I was diagnosed. This was a way in which he could become more independent and help alleviate a chore that took up too much of my energy during treatment. As he grew up, I have had countless conversations with him regarding either the need to do his laundry, get his clothes out of the dryer, or just pick up the clothes off of his floor so that I could remember the color of the carpet. During his junior year of high school, I could see how overwhelmed he was with studying for his advanced placement classes and that his stress was mounting to an unprecedented level. I walked into his room, ready to lay into him about the clothes on his floor, when I realized that this was actually a chance for me to serve him. For him to see that I see his hard work and I see his stress. He left that Saturday for a study session and came home to all of his clothes laundered and put away. He gave me a huge hug when he came home. The world was piling rocks on his shoulders and I had just lifted one off of him, regardless of how small it might have been. I could have nagged him, but I chose to serve him.

Wouldn't we all love to have others anticipating our needs? Imagine if you spent this week looking at the people around you, anticipating their needs. Imagine how serving someone else would center you in a place of gratitude for how you can use your gifts. But remember that this is an exercise in service and gratitude, not a chance to start keeping score. You do not serve so that someone else will serve you. Anticipating someone else's needs is not always easy. If you come from a place of judgment, you might very well choose to serve them in a way that has a negative connotation to that person. You serve as a way to walk alongside another person wherever they are in their journey.

To be able to be ridiculously present, volunstars disconnect from their phones and social media during the day.

Disconnecting from cell phones can seem like torture for many. We live in an on-demand society where individuals freak out if they are not texted back quickly or we do not answer their emails promptly. This is all a false sense of worth. The more we let others know that we are not comfortable being on demand, the easier it is. I have had an employee that will text me and if I don't text her back on her timeframe, will follow up with an "are we OK?" text. And then possibly another one telling me that she needs an answer. I get it. I get how the rest of the world wants us to be on demand. But we can choose to limit this way more than most people currently are. I understand as a parent that we want to be in contact with our children in case of an emergency. But ask yourself, when was the last text from my child that was an actual emergency? A real emergency! Not them needing an answer to an inane question on their timetable, but a real emergency.

This aspect of our lives requires us to set boundaries that others might not be comfortable with, but they are necessary to move to a place of being ridiculously present.

I have now informed my staff that they are not to text me unless it is an emergency and needs to be answered for the sustainability of the company. I have informed them that I will answer emails once in the morning and once at the end of the day. I have informed them that they should schedule blocks of time for meetings with me when I travel, as opposed to random calls throughout the day. And guess what? It works. I have changed the on-demand expectation. It isn't going to happen unless you change it.

I understand that I am in a position of authority in my company and you might be saying, "My boss would never go for that." What are they willing to do? Have you ever even thought about the parameters that you could ask for?

I am also a parent, so I understand that children don't really like to listen to the boundaries that we try to set. The most annoying parenting experience used to happen when I would take my son to the McDonald's playground. Inevitably, there would be a parent who would threaten their child over and over again. "If you hit him one more time, we are leaving." After hearing that for the fifth time, I wanted to yank their kid out of the play structure and tell them that it was time to make good on their promise of leaving. Setting boundaries with your children is very difficult, but it takes consistency.

Every retreat week, there is an empowering activity on the schedule, designed to have families learn more about themselves.

Little Pink has done hang-gliding, stand-up paddle boarding, knocker ball, parasailing, and more. All of these activities are designed to put participants in a place that is out of their comfort zone, so that they can feel a sense of empowerment, purpose, or renewed energy. I am not advocating for you to turn your life into an extreme adventure sport competition. Rather, how can you change aspects of your life that move you out of your comfort zone so that you can start to see a different perspective, helping you to be able to become more ridiculously present for others? Could you spend 30 minutes a day at a disadvantaged school reading to low-level readers? Could you schedule a class that helps you become centered in your own life? Could you teach someone else a skill that you possess? Could you offer up your services to a person in need? Do you have the ability to choose to invest in yourself in a way that you never imagined?

During every retreat week, a special date night or adult night out is scheduled. The volunstars watch the kids and the adults get to connect.

This is a special time on a retreat because it creates an intimate space for parents and a bonding experience for the children. In short, to be ridiculously present with your significant other, you have to start by at least scheduling time to be present. Growing up in a family with six kids, I rarely remember my parents going out to dinner, unless we were traveling. But they made it crystal clear to us that they were going to prioritize each other. Every night after dinner, the table was cleared and they would shoo everyone out of the kitchen and retreat to the back porch for their 10 minutes of time together. All of us played sports and had extracurricular schedules, creating a matrix of complicated transportation issues, but regardless of that fact, they always got their 10 minutes. Those 10 minutes were torture for the rest of us. We were not allowed to interrupt. If we needed something, we had to wait. It was the longest 10 minutes of our daily lives. The time seemed to pass like molasses through a sieve. We watched them prioritize being ridiculously present with each other and it was an example of how to love your spouse that each of us took away in our adult lives. They didn't have a babysitter, they probably struggled to go out and pay for a fancy dinner and they didn't need to. They found their way of being ridiculously present for each other. My husband and I started doing this when our son was little and it drove him nuts to not be included, making it all the more important. Our children need to see that for relationships to grow and be valued in our lives that we have to prioritize them.

Every meal begins with a prayer and the seating arrangement is set up to maximize people getting to know each other.

It is simple, but it is a way to set the stage for focusing on gratitude. Eat dinner as a family whenever possible. Sit around a table, not a television. Talk about what you are grateful for during the day. Model for your children what appropriate behavior is acceptable at the table. And most importantly, try not to put your judgment wall up so that you are capable of seeing their pain, their excitement, or their changing heart. As parents, we are quick to look at our children as a reflection of ourselves. But they are a reflection of God, not us. On a daily basis, we should focus on how we can be ridiculously present in their lives to help them realize the gifts that God has bestowed upon them. If we are busy molding them into who we want them to be, we are limiting the ability for them to see who God wants them to be. We do not get to choose their profession, their college, and their friends. Rather we help guide them to understanding how their decisions will impact their lives. We offer them a strong foundation of how God loves them. We serve them in their pain and brokenness and we find a way every day to make being ridiculously present in their lives one of our greatest priorities.

I was a senior in high school when my father's company reassigned him to a plant in South Carolina, which would not have been an easy bus ride every morning from Pennsylvania. I had been a standout basketball and field hockey player, and the thought of moving was difficult to comprehend. My family had moved many times, so we knew as children that we did not really have a say in the decision-making. My dad decided that he would commute back and forth to South Carolina so that I could finish out my senior year and hopefully get a college scholarship. I am sure that this was a difficult decision for him and my mother to make, one they did not take lightly. But what I remember vividly was at every single field hockey game, basketball game, school awards ceremony, prom and more, when I looked up, my dad was always there. He was there with his smile, hugs, and would talk to me about every aspect of my life. He had made the decision to have it be hard on him, rather than me. He decided that the only way to be ridiculously present in my life was to be present. What a gift to me! I look back at the sacrifices that my parents made and those are the lessons that help me to put the concept of parenting in perspective. Parenting is an ongoing exercise in sacrifice. You will find yourself needing to sacrifice something in your life to be ridiculously present with yourself, others, and God. Don't be fooled. It is a decision that has opportunity costs. It is a decision with abundant grace as the reward.

Families typically comment how amazing it is to have a week where they do not have to think about what to prepare for dinner and get to just follow a schedule.

Families show up and everything is taken care of for them. Obviously, this makes being ridiculously present with each other an easier task. But think about your everyday life and how making small changes can help you prioritize being ridiculously present with the people that you love. Maybe you can have one of your children be your special dinner helper. What a great chance to help them become more responsible, but also create an environment where you can get to know their heart better. Maybe you have a resistant teenager who comes home and shuts himself in his room and plays video games all afternoon. It seems hopeless. The wall is up and it is solid brick. You wonder how to fix him. Realize that is the wrong question. How can you serve him?

Maybe it is a matter of asking if he will teach you to play a certain game. Show up, don't give up. Think of every part of our life as just a blip on the radar. Be a consistent pattern of light on the radar, not just a shooting star in the sky.

We ask our families to reflect on the week and write a letter.

The outpouring of love during the week can be very overwhelming for many families. Complete strangers have given their time, resources, and talents to care for their family. Many families seem like they can barely catch a breath when they arrive, yet leave ready for their battle and united as a family. We never want them to leave without processing the week. We conduct a final meeting where they answer the question, "What was the best part of your week?" We share the experience in the volunstar house during the week and let them know that each night we have committed to this practice and that each and everyone of them has been a part of one of the volunstar's best parts of their days.

Each of our final nights with this meeting is something that is emotional, awe inspiring, and contains an immeasurable level of commitment to the people they love. To watch grown men discuss how the week provided them a chance to put their family first, or that they have been struggling as a couple and have rekindled their love, or that the bond they created with the other guys going through the same thing are friendships for life, is moving. To hear the children speak of the bravery of their moms in a way that you can tell they have never verbalized, or the friendships they have created and their plans to visit each other, will warm your heart. The cancer survivors discuss how they came as complete strangers and are leaving as family. They express how rewarding it is to have the chance for their families to be cared for and the guilt that they have about being sick and how that has affected the family unit. The night usually contains many tears, tons of laughter, and good-bye hugs that never seem to end.

In our own lives, do we take time to put words to our feelings? Part of being ridiculously present is reflecting on our lives and our relationships and putting words to them, either written or verbal, so that others know how we feel. Start telling people what they mean to you right now. Send them a text, a card, or call them. Do not let another minute go by without every day being a chance to let people know how you feel. It is liberating to engage in an authentic life of open honesty. This is how you will be true to yourself and start to see your ability to impact others through your actions. You will also start to realize, when you become vulnerable with your words and truly state what you are feeling, that others will do the same. It is in this deepening of a relationship where authentic friendships and love will develop. It is in this place of vulnerability where you will find it easier to talk and hear God's voice.

Our retreats are not rocket science, but they are lessons in the power of being ridiculously present. To become ridiculously present with others and with God, you will need to become an authentic person that lives with intentionality.

What steps of intentionality can you make that will add value to your life?

How would that decision add quality time to be ridiculously present in other parts of your life change your day?

How can you look at the mundane aspects (carpool, work, chores, etc.) of your life become opportunities to be ridiculously present with others?

Choose the six most important people in your life. Make a decision to have a conversation with them about what they mean to you.

Chapter 19

And what happens if there is only silence? What happens if no matter how hard you are trying, you feel like you never hear God? There are numerous parables about individuals who have been devoutly waiting for God, only to miss Him because they were focused on their version of how He would appear.

> There is a parable of a man who is faced with his home flooding. He prayed to God to save him. His neighbor drives by in his truck and offers the man a ride to safety. The man tells his neighbor that he is confident that God will save him. A boat passes as the waters are rising and offers him help. He refuses because he knows that God will save him. The water rises and the man climbs to the roof of his house when a helicopter spots him and offers him rescue. He declines the offer and looks to the heavens and prays. He eventually perishes and upon standing in front of God, asks Him, "Why didn't you save me?" Of course, God responds, "I sent a truck, a boat, and a helicopter, what more did you want me to do?"

One of the mistakes that many people make is that they are waiting for God to show up in a way that makes sense to them. They may have prayed for God to call them to know how to fit into and serve at their church. But what if God is nudging you to be in the community serving others? While you are waiting for God to dictate your church assignment, you might miss His direction. Maybe you believe that God will find you the perfect job and you grow discontent in your current position, because you have already defined His calling as one that is tied up in your professional career path.

We are incredibly bold when we place parameters on God's plan for our lives.

The silence that we experience is often not really silence, but occurs when our mind and heart are full of our own thoughts and God's voice is being drowned out. I have struggled with this my entire life.

I couldn't hear His voice because I was busy not thinking about what I actually believed.

The constant barrage of thoughts of not being good enough were loud voices and God's was a faint whisper. It took a megaphone for God to get through to me.

But He kept pursuing me.

He never gave up on the path that He had for me. He chose me long before I ever knew it to do this work and I finally let Him catch me. God continues to pursue you. He is not silent. He may be moving other puzzle pieces around to move you to be ready. He might be preparing you in other ways, but He is not silent. You may not be able to hear His call, but can you feel His care? What exists in the silence? In the silence that is where you can start:

Living an authentic life
Living a ridiculously present life

In the absence of hearing Him, you can choose to start living like Him. The church that I attend has been a blessing in my life in so many ways. Partly because I still feel like a flawed and broken person and am truly accepted there. But also because we focus on making Jesus famous. That phrase, "Making Jesus Famous," is one that requires us to live an authentic life. It mandates that we are ridiculously present in the lives of others and with God. When I first visited my pastor to discuss my calling, I remember feeling like I was not good enough because I didn't seem like I knew enough about God. I didn't know Bible verses and I didn't care about reading the Bible. I have realized that making Jesus famous is about recklessly abandoning all of those thoughts and accepting myself where I am. I now look at the Bible for inspiration and direction, not as a chore. I know that God does not expect me to know everything that He has in store, but that I must be willing to be ridiculously present with Him to hear His voice. I also realize that my imperfections offer access for others to see how He can work through a flawed person.

In full disclosure, I struggle to not drop curse words here and there. More here than there. I still judge people in my life and get upset when things don't go my way. I work to keep my marriage vibrant while I travel all over the country. I am challenged by how to grow a company on a national scale without losing its personal touch. I struggle with a son that is becoming more independent, now that he is off at college and doesn't seem to need his mother as much as he used to. I am human. God expects nothing less than that. If I could hang a sign on my chest describing who I am, it would probably say *Work Under Construction*.

I have had numerous people confide to me that they wish that God would clearly show up in their lives like He did in mine on that fateful day on the beach. My response is always that He was showing up in my life for years and years in gentle nudges and sacred echoes, but I was just too stubborn and full of myself to see Him. God is with us all the time. I wasn't looking for Him, I was running away from Him. He chased me and He found me anyway. God is in constant pursuit of each and every one of us. He knows everything about you. What is in the way of letting Him catch you?

God showing up is not the answer.

Being confident that He is already showing up is the key.

Answering His call is only the beginning.

The biggest mistake that I could make would be to think that God called me to create and build Little Pink Houses of Hope and that He is done with me. Check, I answered His call, that's it. On the contrary, my life is now full of intentionality and reflection to create an awareness of how else He wants me to move. I have watched Him do everything that He has done in my life and in the creation of an organization that serves so many. But I am still scared. What might He ask of me next?

Am I ready to be ridiculously present with Him for the next ANYTHING that He asks of me?

What if I do such a good job with what He has asked that I use up my purpose here on Earth—will that be when my cancer comes back? What if I am so wrapped up in the work that I am doing that I don't hear His voice again?

Following God's calling is not a one-time experience.

It is an ongoing journey, with twists and turns that I will not see coming. There is pain and heartbreak waiting for me down the road.

But God is on the road with me.

I have told a few people something that has always been crystal clear to me as well. God called me to breathe life into Little Pink, which does not mean that He called me to be there until the end.

I want to be open to how He can use me, up until my last breath.

What area of your life have you determined is where God's calling for you will be?

Is that question getting in the way of you being open to a greater plan that He might have for you?

How could you begin to "Make Jesus Famous" today?

Chapter 20

Imagine that tomorrow doctors explained to you that you have another 40 years to live. Would you really change that much? The clock would start ticking, but the world would continue around you in a fairly normal fashion. Heck, 40 years might be more than you ever imagined!

Now, imagine that the same doctor told you that you have 10 years. You might choose to put a bucket list together of things that you NEED to do—the artificial list of "things" that, if done, will somehow prove that you have lived. Steps to change your job or spend more time with your family could also be a part of your preparation.

But imagine if you are told that you have just this moment. Then what? You would find yourself not thinking about a bucket list—you would only think about the people that you love or God. You would even gasp that breath in differently. You wouldn't want to miss a single thing.

Life can be filled with curveballs, thrown at us right and left. It might be a cancer diagnosis, a terminal illness, an addiction, or even death. All of these life-changing events act like a magnifying glass on our lives. When the magnifying glass is put up against our relationships, what does it reveal? If a relationship or the way you think about yourself is dysfunctional or broken, the small fissure will look like a deep chasm under the magnifying glass. It can seem as vast as the Grand Canyon. If you had been ridiculously present in that relationship, what would it have looked like under the glass?

In contrast, if there is a strong love present, the magnifying glass can reveal a beauty never thought imaginable. Cancer was my magnifying glass. I had to take stock of my life and all of my relationships. I had to change my entire definition of healing.

When I first got diagnosed, so many people would say, "I will pray for your healing." Others would be so bold as to say, "If you would pray harder, you will be healed." Both of these statements made me want to scream!

So many people think of healing as just a physical aspect or journey, but when you are diagnosed with cancer, for many, healing takes on a whole new meaning. I had only ever thought of healing as a physical sensation until I spoke on the phone with Marie, a participant on our first retreat.

Marie had a unique outlook on healing. It was her view that she could spend all of her time trying to heal herself physically and not be prepared spiritually and emotionally for the end. Or she could do the opposite, focus on her emotional healing and forego treatment that was most likely going to cause her death. Marie came from a family with a rare disease and there was not a single member of her family who had ever lived past the age of 35. Marie was 33. She had found a way to put the experience in perspective in a way that no one had ever presented to me before. She stated that her goal was for a complete healing. A healing that consisted of working on her physical challenges, repairing broken relationships, forging an honesty with God, becoming a wife for her husband of only a year, and healing her soul. Her plan of healing had nothing to do with outcomes that anyone else would be able to see. Healing for Marie was about presenting herself before God as her best, most healed self. She changed the way that I viewed the word "battle" in the cancer community as well. She stated very clearly that she would not lose. Her battle was not one focused on cancer, but healing. She would win the battle of healing and still be victorious, even in her death. She could die and still win the battle of healing. Her healing inspired me up until her very last breath.

During my cancer journey, I was forced into a world of medical advocacy and had to figure out how to navigate the medical jargon to be able to even have a chance at physical healing. There was no one in the medical community that will ever care as much as I did about my care and the outcome of whether I lived or died.

But on that same journey, I realized that healing is more than just the physical journey. I was lucky enough to have the epiphany that I got the do-over. The chance to work on healing all aspects of my life if I could just become ridiculously present and engaged in my life.

Physical healing can seem overwhelming. Sometimes, physical healing is not meant to be. Individuals can work to try to make their body conducive to healing, but the end result might still be the same. Often, individuals have developed patterns of living that make it hard to see how physical healing can happen. On a recent retreat, a participant got off the ferryboat with walker in hand. Walking from the dock to the car was a chore for her. She was 43 years old and using a walker. She could not remember the last time she actually left her house to go to something other than a doctor's visit, and now she found herself on a Caribbean Island and was nervous. Her world at home consisted of going from her bed to the bathroom or the kitchen. She was with her husband, who was at her beck and call. When she arrived and walked into her bedroom, she started crying when she saw the beautiful view of the Caribbean. She told me that she spent every day in her bed at home staring at a ceiling fan, and that this view was amazing.

The first night when retreat participants met and introduced themselves, she focused on everything that was wrong in her life. Money was a struggle, kids that didn't visit enough broke her heart, and a disease that caused her tons of agony dominated her life. During the retreat week, our volunstars focus on serving in a way that focuses the participants on embracing the life that they have. I could see a spring start to appear in her step. Throughout the week, she proceeded to walk more than she had in the entire previous year. She snorkeled, she danced, and became affectionate with her husband. She started to heal mentally and it was manifesting itself as a physical healing. She was changing her view of herself from victim to survivor. At the end of the week, she was ready to throw her walker into the Caribbean Sea.

When we focus on healing spiritually, we are putting time and energy into becoming our best self. We seek out peace and comfort and try to find a way to put our trust in God.

Spiritual healing is only possible by being authentic and reflective.

On another family retreat, I had a mother come up to me on the third day to say that her daughter kept asking them about the prayers that we said prior to each meal. She had asked her mother why her family didn't pray. The mother came to me very tongue-in-cheek and said I was getting them in trouble as parents. There is no pressure of any kind on our retreats, regardless of religious background. We openly support all faiths and encourage people of other faiths to share their customs, prayers, and holiday traditions when they fall in a retreat week. As an organization, we can't be ridiculously present if we do not acknowledge and celebrate other people's faith. The mother came to me at the end of the week and said that it had been a long time since her and her husband had attended synagogue, but this week, being pushed by their daughter had caused the conversation to come up again. They left the retreat week and it was months before I heard back from her.

When she called me, it was not with good news. Her cancer had spread and they were struggling to get it under control. And then she told me why she was calling.

She wanted to thank me for all of the times that we had prayed. She and her husband went home and started going back to synagogue. She stated that her spiritual awakening was the only way in which she could imagine being able to process the end drawing near. She couldn't imagine her own daughter not being exposed to what a conversation with God could look like in her life. She knew that in the coming months, her daughter would need to turn to God and she was thankful that she had been there to witness her spiritual growth alongside her daughter. She was thanking me for the one thing that I was petrified to do when I started the organization—be a spiritual leader.

I meet with a spiritual mentor who leads and guides me so that I will continue to develop my relationship with God and better understand His Word. She never makes me feel like I have to be someone that I am not. And in the end, I know that she is one of the people that God put in my path to remind me that I am good enough.

Because I believe that is what God does. He puts people in our path because we are on a journey. He doesn't expect each of us to start in the same spot or move at the same pace. He requires the simple giving of our hearts to Him for the journey to begin.

What is the curveball in your life that you have been thrown?

When you look under the magnifying glass, what do you see?

Chapter 21

Healing relationships is often one of the hardest forms of healing. It is not something that we can do quietly in our heads. It most often requires us to have critical conversations with people in our lives or subject ourselves to the harsh and destructive reality of who we may have let in. The shortened time frame of a life-altering event gives you a sense of urgency for forgiveness, healing, and love but it can only come in a place of being ridiculously present.

One of my favorite families to attend a retreat almost did not.

Angela and her husband had separated and were living apart when they got their notification that they had been accepted into a retreat week. They had already decided that they would get divorced. They decided that this would be a final family trip, not to heal any divisions between them, just as a gift to their two beautiful children. Their distance throughout the week slowly narrowed. Their growing love was evident to the entire volunstar group. On the very last night, they stood up and told their story. They talked about having a chance to not focus on making dinner and busy parenting tasks like carpooling, but when everything else was stripped away, that they saw each other again for the first time. They realized that everything that they needed they had in each other.

They had healed their relationship by being ridiculously present with each other and putting that above all else. That week was a restart button for their marriage.

Relationships can change if we pour ourselves into them with reckless abandon!

When we focus on healing ourselves emotionally, we are working on rewriting the stories that we tell ourselves. We put time and energy into releasing the hurt and pain of our past. Emotional healing allows individuals to change the negative thinking to positive talk and a positive attitude is an important aspect of braving the harrowing waters of the life changing experiences that are thrust upon us.

Emotional healing will not happen without a decision to give it time and attention.

Breast cancer patients, over and over again, at the age of 28, 32, and 35 attend our retreats and then they pass away. I still want to scream. They are way too young. Patients with kids and spouses, on the cusp of actually starting their life, not having it come to an end. The question that I get more than any other question is: How do I handle all of the death? How do I deal with so many participants that we serve pass away and not go insane? The truth is that it is hard.

It has become somewhat cliché to say that when one person is diagnosed in a family, the whole family is affected. Well, yes, of course. But what it really means is that deep inside each person, there are hurts, pains, and aspects of their lives that have changed. When these changes go unrecognized, the feeling can compound. Those who have married have all stood up with some version of "in sickness and in health, for richer or for poorer, till death do us part." But we don't imagine that the sickness will ravage the person's body, their spirit, and their mental capabilities. We can't foresee that just getting basic cancer treatment can financially destroy a family. We don't imagine that the death part will happen at such a young age, leaving a widow with three small kids. We naively say the words, hope for the best, and pray that it is not us. We don't imagine that His call might not be what we want for our lives. We don't imagine being too proud, broken, or hurt to say yes.

On September 23, 2010, I was sitting in the chemo chair at the hospital for the last time when my mom called to say that my dad had been diagnosed with bladder cancer. I rushed from Duke University's infusion room in North Carolina to their home in Florida without even thinking about my own well-being. Out of thin air, my dad had gone from a vibrant doting father to an invalid overnight due to medical complications. My dad lasted four additional months before he passed away. My dad was instrumental in helping develop a business plan for Little Pink Houses of Hope. I was an educator, I knew nothing about how to start a business. As we were working on the plans in the summer of 2010 prior to his diagnosis, my dad made a joke about how he would be my first and last volunteer. He told me that he was all in and would like his nametag to say, "First volunteer." We laughed and I truly enjoyed working on the plan together and seeing his business acumen. As his child, I had rarely thought of him in those terms. He had always just been my dad. In this environment, I could see why he had climbed the corporate ladder of a fortune 500 company and had such great success. His passing at the age of 69 was devastating to me. I was his little girl. I was also saddened by the fact that my "first volunteer" would never see a retreat happen.

In April of 2011, we conducted our first retreat. As the first year of retreats unfolded, it was full of countless blessings. And then December arrived and five retreat participants passed away between December 1 and December 26, 2011. I was already struggling with the thought of the first Christmas without my dad and it all just felt like too much. I had known all of those women. I had seen how much their husbands loved them. I witnessed how desperately their children were blessed by having them in their lives.

I didn't know how I could do this work anymore.

I went to see a therapist. Out of those sessions came an interesting strategy that I have learned to employ in the rest of my life. The therapist talked to me about how I could reframe the experience.

Reframe it? I was pissed off and hurt.

I wanted my dad back and I didn't want to invest my time with all of these new people who were just going to die at some point. And to top it off, in the back of my own mind, I was still worried that I might not make it either.

In our discussions, we circled back to the idea that my dad had of being the first and last volunteer. When he originally made the statement, it had not registered as anything more than the strength of his commitment. I have learned to reframe the experience, so that now, when any of our retreat participants pass away, I envision him greeting each of the deceased in heaven with a big huge hug from their Little Pink family. I look up at the stars on a day when someone passes away and imagine that the stars are pinholes in the sky where the light of their smiles shine through so that I can see they are alright. I had to be ridiculously present with my grief to be able to start to heal emotionally.

There is one central theme around the topic of all aspects of healing—you must become ridiculously present in all aspects of your life to begin the healing process.

And my dad was right. He is the first and last volunteer.

I am sure that God gave him his nametag when he arrived.

What aspects of your life need healing?

What part of your life would benefit most if you focused some time and attention on the healing that needs to happen?

How can you start to believe that God is ridiculously present with you as you heal?

Chapter 22

So many times, cancer patients state, "I never imagined that my cancer diagnosis would actually be a blessing or a gift." Typically, it is phrased a little harsher, like, "Having cancer sucks, but so much good has come out of it."

People might hear that and not understand. How can a tragedy be a gift?

I started to understand that I was living now as part of the journey of dying. Death is scary. Death is scary because we worry about the people that we leave behind. Death is inevitable. The antidote is when living becomes more beautiful, more full of color and laughter, and feeling. It doesn't take the fear of death away, it makes a person understand how much life is truly a gift! It isn't a gift that is measured in minutes or days, but measured in engagement.

The most rewarding, amazing, and fulfilling time of your life can come when you are ridiculously present, and act upon living an engaged life.

My least favorite thing that people say to me and other cancer patients is a metaphor, which I am sure, is designed to show that they understand, but in the end, highlights how little they know about having cancer. I have heard it time and time again. A cancer patient says that he or she has a fear of dying and a person says, "We could all die at any time—anyone could be hit by a bus tomorrow," in response.

I think that this is a hysterical statement, considering I live in a small town without bus service. If a bus actually hit me, it would probably be a pretty big story. For cancer patients and terminally ill patients, here is the reality:

The bus has already hit us.

For some of us, we got scraped, and when we see a bus, it causes our stomach to get weak, thinking that it might hit us again. We have bus post-traumatic stress disorder. Others are still being dragged under the bus every day. Those people can see the underside of the bus. They have a view of the axle, gears, and the brakes. If only the brakes would stop this bus. If you have never been hit by this bus, you don't know the feeling that the entire rest of your life might be one long bus ride. You'll be scraped and battered along the way and have no chance of ever pulling the cord to let the driver know that you want off the bus.

Even when being dragged under the bus, there is a realization that regardless of what is happening, you are still moving. You might physically look beaten and bruised, but your heart also looks different. You might not have as much energy as you used to, but life is now an exercise in learning to give your energy to the people who matter the most.

Cancer was my bus. I physically look different after the ride. I emotionally shed enough tears to have the windshield wipers on high gear during most of the ride.

But I learned who was driving the bus.

God was going to make sure that if I was bruised and battered, I was loved. If I felt alone on the bus, He put other people in the seats next to me to provide comfort. And when it felt like I could not take another minute on the bus, He opened up the windows and doors and let His radiant sunshine shine upon me.

And then He told me to get off the bus at the ANYTHING stop and get busy!

I have learned that people will come into my life that have been hurt worse than I can ever imagine. Others come and I have a chance to comfort them, while others will not make it. Don't wait for the bus to hit you. Decide to be ridiculously present in the lives of everyone you meet. Grab a front row seat. You will have the best view of the people that you love. You will realize that you can care for them even in your own brokenness. I didn't choose cancer. I didn't choose the circumstances that brought me to my knees—but I am the only one that gets to choose to be ridiculously present in the lives of everyone around me.

Do you have a tragedy in your life that you were able to see as a possible gift?

If you were hit by a tragedy bus, how do you think your thinking would change?

You don't have to wait for the bus to hit you. You have the ability to change right now.

Chapter 23

During our life, we have a chance to hit the restart button, over and over again. This is a chance to redefine our priorities so that we can be ridiculously present and make Him famous. This is your chance to prove that Good Enough is never enough when an abundant life in God's love is what you are destined for.

Making the decision to answer His call was the beginning of Little Pink Houses of Hope, but more importantly it was the beginning of really putting my faith in action. It was the beginning of a relationship that I had deep down always yearned for, but did not know how to achieve. I made tons of mistakes along the way, but I chose to rest in His care. He did not expect perfection. In fact, I think that I enjoy the moments when I am at my lowest and something happens that takes my breath away. In the past, I would have written it off as a coincidence. Now I clearly see it as God making sure that I know that He is still paying attention. He is letting me know, I have not forgotten about you.

You are my child, I think about you constantly and only want the best for you.

His vision on the beach that day was clear. *Create a place for cancer patients to come and be loved.* I was struck by God's hope for my life that day. The hamster in my brain took off and has continued running on His wheel at warp speed. Through the year and a half of treatment, numerous support group meetings, national conferences that I attended and just plain common sense, He caused me to see that the family unit needs additional care and attention while a person is going through treatment. He created an understanding in my heart that I must change and become a person who is ridiculously present in the lives of others to do His work. He has cared for me by putting the right people in my path along the way. None of this is coincidence.

It is the story that He has written that I am lucky enough to be a character in.

There is a universal lesson in my story. We are all broken and flawed in some way. God has not given up on us even though we may have given up on Him. He is in constant pursuit of us. We can choose to be ridiculously present in the lives of others and our universe will open up to experiences we never imagined. We each breathe in and out thousands of times each day. Every breath is a chance to keep doing things exactly the same and letting insecurities about worth dominate our thoughts. Or, we can choose to have every breath be one that is given over to God, so He can breathe His purpose into us. We can be His hands and feet here on Earth. We can do ANYTHING that He asks.

So what is holding you back from being ridiculously present in your life and your relationship with God?

Where are you in your life? Are you just going through the motions? Are you in a bargaining place with God?

What would happen if you were vulnerable in your prayer life? Imagine talking to God about your struggles, your fears, and your deepest dreams of how to answer His call. And then become ridiculously present with Him in your heart.

He is nudging you.

He is putting people in your path.

He is surrounding you with His love.

He is with you in the darkness and your worst moments.

Don't make Him into what you need Him to be. Trust Him and let God be God.

Become present with Him in the Word.
Become present with Him in community.
Become present with Him in your relationships.
Become present with Him in your brokenness.
Become present with Him in your joy.
Become ridiculously present in His love.

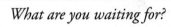

What are you waiting for?

Acknowledgments

In a world that is hurried and rushed, there was only one way for me to write this book. I had to leave my usual surroundings and become ridiculously present with the message before me. I could not have completed this book without the gift of a beautiful place to write at the beach from Paula Lowe and Kate Weiss. The gift of your homes gave me the peace and solitude to tap into the hard words, the silly stories, and the ability to connect with God during the writing process.

When I felt compelled to write this book, I also became incredibly scared. It is not easy to look at the good, the bad, the ugly and actually write it on paper. Along the way, many people who believed in me encouraged me to finish this book so that its message could help others. I am so thankful for Suzanne Smith for saying yes to helping make this book possible so that a large percentage of the proceeds can go to Little Pink. God is working through our friendship and it is a delight to see where he is taking us! I have also had a very close-knit group of friends read, edit, comment and give me their honest reactions—all of which improved the final manuscript.

As a first-time author, I would like to thank the Front Edge Publishing crew for publishing my book, encouraging me and believing in the words and vision of what we have accomplished together.

It has always been crystal clear to me that I have been very lucky to have such a strong and supportive family. To each of my brothers and sisters and sisters-in-law: Your belief in this crazy orbit that I spin in and your willingness to be a part of it makes my heart practically explode. This book is about being ridiculously present and I thank each of you for showing up and being present all the time in my life! We are only able to be this way because of the wonderful example of our beautiful parents. Although my father passed away years ago, my mother's example of continuously living and embracing life with a smile is a total inspiration. The gift of family is and should never taken for granted.

There are so many wonderful friends who have encouraged and inspired me; friends who have cried with me; and friends that have helped with a glass of wine or a shoulder to cry on. To each of them, I want to acknowledge how you have helped me always feel like a member of a fun tribe as opposed to a person stranded on an island alone. The way in which you have accepted me for exactly who I am allows real and authentic relationships, which I cherish and hold close to my heart.

To the many families and volunteers who have attended a Little Pink retreat throughout the years: Your stories, gratefulness, love and connectedness have opened my life up and filled me with immense joy. Our time together matters and it becomes a part of why I choose to continue to love and move forward to grow the organization. I tell people all the time that I have the best job in the world and it is because I have a front row seat to the goodness that exists in the world.

To our amazing staff and board of directors: You have become such wonderful friends! I know that each of you loves this journey as much as I do. Together, we mourn participants who pass away—and celebrate with families as they are accepted into our retreats. Thank you for sharing your love and compassion on this amazing journey with me.

Most importantly, I have to thank my dear husband Terry and son, Jake. Since the very beginning, you encouraged me and celebrated this effort, even when this work has included additional time away. In a world where hope is a key essential ingredient for the work that I do, you make me feel like there is a reason for hope to exist. This journey has not always been easy, but together, we are creating a beautiful legacy. Your love is what fills my heart up and allows me to give so much of myself away to others because I know that you will always be there to refill my well. We have been through so much together as a family and I am the luckiest girl in the whole wide world to bask in your love.

About the Author

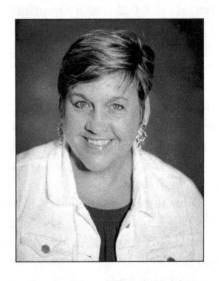

Jeanine Patten-Coble was a high school history teacher and professional educational trainer for 15 years before being diagnosed with breast cancer in 2009. Her own battle with breast cancer inspired the creation of Little Pink Houses of Hope– a nonprofit organization that provides breast cancer survivors and their families a free week long, fun-filled vacation with other families on the breast cancer journey. Jeanine lives in North Carolina with her wonderful husband, Terry, and son, Jake who carried her through her own cancer journey with their strength, support, and love. She continues to be amazed and inspired by all of the wonderful people that she has met through her service and is thankful that God showed up in her life in such a big and powerful way to put her on this mission.

Call to Action

If this book has prompted you to become ridiculously present in your own life or the lives of others, I am thrilled.

Get started today! Don't wait until next week or next month. Jump in now!

Find an organization that sparks your passion and get involved. If you want to become a part of our nonprofit, then I welcome you! Little Pink Houses of Hope offers countless opportunities for people to get involved in directly serving breast-cancer families. From short phone calls to weeklong opportunities for service—and everything in between—our organization can use your gifts and talents. Know that your gifts will be cherished and your heart will become full.

Care to learn more?

Visit www.LittlePink.org or call the office at (336) 213-4733.

CPSIA information can be obtained
at www.ICGtesting.com
Printed in the USA
BVHW071426040821
613449BV00004B/437